Nancy's Journey

A Feisty Cancer Story

Nancy Lofstead

Nancy Lofstead (signature)

Dana Hills Press
Morgantown, West Virginia

ISBN: 0-9712471-0-2
LCCN: 132811

Design by *Angela Caudill*.

The photo on the back cover was taken by my dad, Richard Satterfield. He shot it during a summer outing at Coopers Rock State Forest near my home in Morgantown, West Virginia. The Forest is a place I have been visiting with my family since I was a small child. It continues to provide both an escape and a fascination for me with its giant rock outcrops, dense green hillsides and centuries-old trees. —*N.L.*

Dedication

to *Dave*
my husband, lover and best friend,
who gives me strength and inspiration
along the winding path of this journey.

A Special Note of Gratitude...

to *Mom,*
who supported me with her love, prayers
and encouragement
throughout my years of struggle
despite battling her own crippling illness.

to *Dad,*
who continues to inspire me
through his own example
about the importance of attitude and perseverance
in conquering life's challenges.

Acknowledgments

There are so many people I must consider when it comes to thanking those who have helped me produce the story of my life with cancer. Along the way, close friends, relatives and even casual acquaintances have urged me to record my experiences. In some way or another, either directly or indirectly, the individuals I mention here have played a role in the evolution of this book and deserve my heartfelt gratitude.

My son Greg, his wife Jill and their son, Ethan.

My son Geoff and his wife Tricia.

My three special sisters, Linda, Judy and Carla and my brother D.L.

My other family members: Lee, Kathi, Eric, Christopher, Zachary and Matthew. Jim, Mike, Terri, Kevin, Brent and Aimme. Lolli, Todd, Kristi, Kayla. John, Nicole, Michael, Natalie, and Ronny. Dan, Becky, Macall, Chris and Diana. Bette, Dave, Bryan and Masina. Grandma Stout. Gerald and Gloria.

Ben, Aggie, Great-Aunt Emma. Their sacrifices forced me to acknowledge the selective nature of cancer. As an eyewitness to their suffering, I gained an intimate perspective on the powerful grip of this disease well before the onset of my illness.

—the boundless love of my family helped me set and then accomplish the goal of publishing this book.

I thank my minister, Rev. Daniel Agnew, his wife Ruby, and my entire church family from Harner Chapel United Methodist Church, for all of their prayers and outreach. Their faith gives me strength on an ongoing basis, and has affirmed my desire to create this book.

My friend Ellyn Parsons pushed me to get moving on the task of making this work a reality. Her strong encouragement and the introduction she provided to Populore Publishing Company was the starting point. Populore's professional services were invaluable in my quest to self-publish.

Populore owner Rae Jean Sielen has skillfully shepherded and overseen my book project from start to finish. From the beginning, her vision and belief in my purpose were clearly present as she organized the timeline and executed the production of *Nancy's Journey.* She has always been kind and supportive and has earned my deep respect for her expertise and conscientiousness. I am so appreciative of her confidence in my story's book worthiness.

Bonnie Brown has provided superb editorial services with her competent, compassionate and detail-oriented approach. Her keen memory and listening skills helped me describe more than twelve years of my life with precision and clarity. Bonnie is attentive, responsive and really understood what I wanted to communicate. A special note—I will always believe it was fate and not mere coincidence that brought Bonnie to this project. During the process of helping me produce this book, she showed great empathy toward me. This was due in part to her recent pregnancy-related illness and her encounter with some of the very medical symptoms I've endured over the years. She underwent some of the same hospital procedures and had even taken some of the same medications! Her dedication to the project was evident when she took time to consult with me even while she was feeling the discomfort of late pregnancy—to the point that we met in her hospital room just days before the delivery of her baby son!

Angela Caudill, who designed the book and pulled it all together to create an attractive presentation in both cover and text.

Denise Massie, who, many years ago, encouraged me to record my thoughts and keep records for the ultimate compilation of this work. I'm grateful for her typed transcripts of my initial recollections, which provided a seed for the larger project. I also thank Barb Leonard who generously transcribed tapes during my early efforts to start the book.

"Relay for Life" organizers and participants, especially the American Cancer Society.

My "cancer cousins," whose hard-fought battles against our common enemy are an inspiration to all of us.

Along with their oncologists, I appreciate cancer patients everywhere, whose presence in the world reminds us all about the frailty of our existence as we share the collective human experience. In addition, I wish to thank the many scientists and researchers whose life's work has produced the foundation of care and treatment for cancer patients.

Those who supported me with their love, kindnesses, encouragement and prayers...

All of my co-workers at HealthWorks and MPTA (who created a circle of support, which helped buoy me when I felt as though I would fall), the GE Specialty Chemicals family, Linda Manley, Julie Lattanzi, Nicole Bakos, Linda Vaji, Jack and Carol Brautigam, Barb Leonard, Linda and Scot Anderson, Charlie and Loretta Florence, Jan and Mike Malone, Jerry and Pam Burgess, the Bill Baron family, Joe Merandino, Mitch and Karen Spengler, Bonnie and Dan Meadows, Joanna Luckey, Susan Rhodes, Lisa Lewandowski, Mike and Julie Parsons, John and Sabra Spiker, Jeff and Debbie Benson, Craig and Nancy Walker, Ray and Jane Stiles, Bonnie Fox, Dan and Connie Erenrich, Dave "Sugar" Walls, Cynthia "Sam" Booth, Annetta Haddox, Mark and Kathy Beckett, Kevin and Carrie Bastin, Drew and Lori Shea, Tom Colt, Merry Ann Nehlen, Rudy and Helen Almasy, Fred and Glenna Wells, Tom and Sue Hall, Carl and Maxine Wise, Liz and Pat Zuchowski, Nana Rogers, Dennis and Nancy Porter, Jodi and Karl Novak, Linda and Luis Orteza, Bill and Debbie Dean, Melinda Shrout, Dorothy Stoll, Pete Zulia, Doug Patch, Jim and Donna Lattanzi, Betty Vanscoy, Patty Liberatore, Helen Shearer, Rose and George Saunders, Alex Matlins, Liz Fleeson, Emily and Terry Jones, Mick and Sue Carlock, Kent Manley, Linda and Okey DeWitt, Art and Rhea Wilson, Brenda Quertinmont, Lori and Richie Martin, John and Heather Throckmorton, Jane Riffe, Kevin and Pam Workman, Frank and Nancy McGreevy, Fred and Peg Wotring, Kelly Simons, Joy Boguszewski, Patty Arnold, Dorothy Saunders, John and Polly Kovalchek, Janna Ott, Margaret Carpenter, Bill and Carol Kling, Barb Haller, Bob and Jeanne Moore, Frank Moore, Chris Ryan, Jim and Carol Craig, Bill and Carolyn Ryan, Bob and Connie Meadows, Pat Malott, Lynn Matthews, Mary Nuce, Dan and Joyce Payne, Carolyn McBee, Laura Westerman, Sandy Amandus, Pat Harper, Ann Ridings, Chris and Amy Rivell, Dorothy Rowan, Betty Puskar, Joy Saab, Regina Chico, Rick Stache and the staff at Richard Bradley Salon, Terry and Marty Sippin, Loretta and George Sanders, Julia Tenney, Jim and Moira Tippy, Carolyn Haskiell, Joyce and Darrell Hardman, Bill and Vicki Hawley, Jerri Eskew, Mary Dale Brown, Sally Wilson, Deb Sanders,

Janice Goodwin, Tim and Lourene Reed, Allen Kerns, Joan Selby, John DeBlasis, Bob and Jan Cox, June Lloyd, Doug and Judy Harman, Elaine Zalar, Nancy Lilly, Joyce Landacre, Zach Spiker, Tim Spiker, Rev. Robert Scott Dixon, Carol Ramsburg, Dave and Cindy Deem, Martha Hupp, Jan Anderson, Kitty Nutter, Jane Pertko, Freda Neely, Allen, Charlotte and Grace at City Office Supply, my friends at Forks of Cheat Baptist Church, including a special thanks to all of the church congregations that continue to remember me in their prayers.

I am grateful to my medical caregivers (doctors, nurses, pathologists, pharmacists, radiologists, receptionists, schedulers, etc.) who have helped me maintain the strength I've needed to stay on task and supplied verification of certain medical terms and references...

A sincere thanks for the T.L.C. from the nurses and medical staff who have cared for (tolerated) me over the years, including Melanie, Rainey, Londia, Katrina, Beth, Angie, Kathy, Sylvia, Tammy, Dorothy, Wenda, Helen, Jean, Lavora, Barb, Lynn, Nancy, Trudy, Faye, Marilyn, Dotsie, Mary, Susan, Carolyn, the 6th Floor chemo nurses at Mon General Hospital (in particular Kim, Vicki, Henrietta, Trish, Kathy, Rachael) and the countless others who have provided support and care.

I also appreciate my physicians, who allowed me to participate in my own health care: Dr. Fouad "George" Abbas, Dr. Miklos Auber, Dr. Elliot Chideckel, Dr. John Currie, Dr. Andrew Heiskell, Dr. Charlene Horan, Dr. Roger King, Dr. Rodney Kovach, Dr. Paul Malone, Dr. Darrell Saunders, Dr. Roy Stevens, and Dr. David Stoll.

I wish to add a special acknowledgment for the care received at the following: The Johns Hopkins Hospital and Clinics, Monongalia General Hospital, Sinai Hospital of Baltimore, West Virginia University Hospitals (including the Mary Babb Randolph Cancer Center and Betty Puskar Breast Care Center).

❦

Finally, and most importantly, I thank God for His constant, abundant blessings and for the strength and courage to continue fighting the battle, and for giving me the opportunity to glorify Him!

Preface

When I first conceived of publishing a work to reflect my experience in the battle against cancer, I imagined a small pamphlet or brochure focusing on the lighter side of how to survive. I pictured writing some little tips I'd picked up over the years and a few tongue-in-cheek suggestions thrown in for good measure (to help emphasize the importance of humor). I could see the publication including an itemized list of simple how-to's, including basic steps for buying a wig and avoiding wicker wastebaskets when nausea sets in.

Instead, I am happy to offer readers this personal, detailed account of my journey with cancer. From the moment of diagnosis in 1989 to the status of my current treatment and ongoing efforts to prolong my survival, I have opened my medical records, my home, and my heart on these pages. However, in order to protect their anonymity, I have not referred to my doctors by name.

Compiling this story was a huge undertaking. From inconsistently jotting down a few anecdotes here and there over the years and losing sight of the project during my emotional "down" periods and bouts of near physical incapacitation, to finally creating a file and recording my stories on tape over the course of several months, my efforts have been a labor of love. Without the help of those around me there may never have been a book.

Throughout these pages are glimpses of the simultaneous pain and joy that cancer has brought to my life. The reader is allowed a view of the whole picture, from shadows that loom around chemo and surgery, to the microscopic truths that have altered my path, to both the physical torture of my cancer and subsequent exhilaration at my body's resilience. It is a testimony to the love that flows in abundance through a life laid bare by disease. My hope is that, in seeing all of these things, others will agree that cancer has been an immeasurable blessing in my life.

My friend Julie Parsons gave me an inspirational reading a few years back. It was titled "Welcome to Holland." In it a woman compares raising a child with special needs to setting out on a trip to Italy and ending up in Holland instead, despite all of her resistance and determination to arrive at the first destination. The author decides the challenge of raising her special child is a blessing she could never have anticipated, just as a twist in travel plans can offer the traveler an entirely new and unexpected trip.

Sometimes I feel like the woman in the story. This journey with cancer is not at all what I had in mind for my life. It's not what I'd pictured for my husband Dave and me and our two sons these last dozen years. But I must admit, it has truly been a beautiful journey.

I present this book as a gift of appreciation to the people whose love has sustained me and whose lives have enlightened me. I also offer it as an essay on hope to others facing the challenge of surviving cancer. If even one patient picks this up and adopts a "take-charge" attitude in directing his or her care, or decides to let go of life's agony and laugh and play instead, I will be gratified.

Lastly, it is my wish that all readers will see the relevance of celebrating survival and value every day with the magnificent reverence life deserves.

Foreword

This Foreword consists of the combined input from two of my most beloved physicians, Dr. John Currie and Dr. Fouad "George" Abbas. I had been Dr. Currie's patient for five years when he left Baltimore for Dartmouth Medical School in New Hampshire in 1995. It was his wish to transfer the care of his patients into the hands of a physician in whom he had complete trust—one whose vast medical expertise was accompanied by immense compassion. With full confidence, he chose Dr. Abbas as his hand-picked successor. —N.L.

Knowing Nancy Lofstead for these many years has been a personal growth experience for me. Life is a mystery and it is the interaction we have with each other that defines its purpose. Through this book I realize that others will be able to share my wonderful experience with Nancy. We all enrich our lives by living with her as she chronicles her struggles. Her wit, enthusiasm and charisma of life are contagious. The uniqueness of each of us is well outlined through her thoughts and reminds us that our character is at the pillar of consciousness. The hearts that are touched with this consciousness is all that we have to count on. She touches me.

Fouad Abbas, M.D.
Director, Division of Gynecologic Oncology
Sinai Hospital of Baltimore

Nancy's Journey: A Feisty Cancer Story fills the heart of the reader with a potpourri of emotional reactions—humor, joy, sadness, pain—all are included in this true story of an amazing woman's fight with the devastations of ovarian cancer. My own reactions were those of fond memories of my part in the story, as the first Baltimore gynecologic oncologist to have the privilege to participate in the care of Nancy Lofstead. As well documented in her story, she embraced every aspect of her disease and its treatment with determination, humor, and realism; while she reacted to good news with expected elation, she and Dave, her stalwart companion and husband, tackled audaciously *every* bit of bad news, treatment changes, or re-operation with a resiliency admixed with humor that was wonderful to participate in as her physician.

Ovarian cancer is a terribly unfair disease; over 25,000 cases are diagnosed annually in the United States, and three fourths of those are advanced when discovered. It seems to have a predilection for attacking productive, creative, and vigorous women in their prime, and when treatment is unsuccessful, it marches to an inevitable robbery of the very vitality that characterized its victims when healthy. Fortunately, however, ovarian cancer *can* be treated successfully and chronically with a persevering oncologist and a willing patient. *Nancy's Journey* documents a penultimate example of such a long battle.

For the gynecologic oncologist, ovarian cancer patients are the ultimate challenge. The surgical management is tedious and dangerous, administration of chemotherapy can be debilitating and risky, and the terrible chore of relating bad news to patients who inevitably become your friends can be overly distressing. Nancy, with her humor, acceptance, and dogged fight, made the journey through her treatment more than just tolerable—I looked forward to seeing her and Dave regardless of the circumstances.

No matter how bad the day, Nancy made it better. It is clear from this book that she affected the lives of family, friends, medical personnel, and other patients in the same way.

John L. Currie, M.D., J.D.
Professor and Chair Emeritus
Department of Obstetrics and Gynecology
Dartmouth Medical School

Contents

CHAPTER 1
In Search of Strength   15

1989 - 1990

CHAPTER 2
Miracles Happen   51

1990 - 1992

CHAPTER 3
Counting My Blessings   71

1994 - 1995

CHAPTER 4
Dance Lessons   107

1996 - 1997

CHAPTER 5
A Celebration Called Life   143

1997 - 2000

CHAPTER 6
Something in the Air   183

2001

Afterword   207

CHAPTER 1

In Search of Strength

1989 - 1990

Words

When I try to remember the first time the word cancer held any real meaning for me, I travel back in time to the late 1960s when I was just a teenager, naïve about both the disease and mortality in general. I can hear the familiar voices of relatives speaking in hushed tones about my great-aunt Emma's breast cancer. I feel afraid, but she wants me to see. She is showing me the scar where her breast had been. I leave her side traumatized by the image.

Aunt Emma lived across the road from my grandmother, her sister. I was close to my aunt and saw her often, except when she began the process of dying. Grandma talked about hearing Emma screaming and moaning in pain. The thought of it scared me and I didn't go to see her when she was in the hospital.

In my experience, cancer wasn't openly talked about at that time. It seemed the word was meant to be whispered. "Isn't it sad about Emma's cancer?" "...such a shame, poor Emma has cancer."

Cancer was not a condition one survived. A diagnosis that included the dreaded word "cancer" meant you were done for. It would be years before I'd make any connection between her fate and mine.

❧

I am an administrative assistant in an outpatient physical therapy clinic in my hometown of Morgantown, West Virginia. I went to work there after our friend John, who was a neighbor, called one day to ask if I'd come over to his clinic and answer the phones and check in patients while he and his wife Sabra were in Hawaii. That was more than twenty years ago. As it happened, the time was right for me to say yes.

My husband Dave and I had agreed that I wouldn't go to work while our two boys were small, but now Greg and Geoff were both in school. And besides, I wanted to add to the one lonesome entry on my resume that dated back to my high school years: hotdog cook at Kelly's Boat Dock, Cheat Lake.

The clinic was a small operation in 1980. The entire staff was comprised of John and me, and one part-time physical therapist. John was teaching at the University then and served as the athletic trainer for the West Virginia University football team, so I was often on my own at the clinic. I was working there in January of 1989 when John approached me about taking a Dale Carnegie self-development course. I wasn't interested.

"I don't want to go. Don't those people have to get up and speak in front of a group?"

He persisted. John said it was the kind of course that would give me more confidence and boost my self-esteem. Ultimately, I gave in and reluctantly marched off to class with Sabra, whom I considered a dear friend, and my co-worker Mark. I struggled through the fourteen-week-long course. Each night we had to go to the front of the room and give a two-minute talk. I'd get up, give my talk (rambling as fast as I could), and run back to my chair, where the sweat poured off every inch of my frame. Asked to choose a specific topic on which to base our talks, I'd picked cancer.

On two occasions I talked about my mother-in-law's treatment for lung cancer. I told about the loss of my nephew Ben, who'd died of neuroblastoma several years earlier. I evolved into an advocate of sorts. I urged my fellow classmates to collect for the American Cancer Society when asked, volunteer for community work, those sorts of things. These were emotional presentations for me. Each time the moral of my story seemed to boil down to, "You never know when someone in your family, a neighbor, or someone close to you will be diagnosed with cancer."

⌘

With every April came my annual visit to the gynecologist. During that particular spring, in 1989, I was having some mild pain on the left side of my abdomen. The doctor didn't think it was anything to worry about, but at my insistence, he scheduled an ultrasound just to give me peace of mind.

Several days after the test, he called with word of a very small cyst on the left ovary.

"The cyst is nothing to be concerned about," he told me over the phone. The second call came a week later, "Your Pap smear was a bit irregular. Better come in and have it repeated."

By the time I went in for the additional Pap, the pain in my side had worsened. So he scheduled a second ultrasound.

"What is THAT? I can see it!" I said to the technician, referring to a huge black area on the monitor screen.

She replied, "Well, we're really not supposed to say anything."

I had to know, "What is it? It looks as big as an egg."

She said the doctor would phone me. His good news/bad news call came a few days later. The follow-up Pap test was negative but the second ultrasound showed the ovarian cyst was getting larger. I'd need to go back in for another appointment.

By now the Dale Carnegie course was winding down. The last class meeting was in early May. A week later, on a Friday, I met with my doctor. His examination proved the cyst was growing. I was feeling a lot of pain. He offered two options: wait three or four months to see what would happen (the cyst could shrink or dissolve on its own) or have a hysterectomy.

The words "borderline potential malignancy" came to mind. I'd heard them pronounced six years earlier with the removal of my right ovary, accepting the situation then as nonchalantly as the threat of rain. Now nearly forty, with no plans for more children, and struggling with problem menstrual periods, I willingly chose the hysterectomy.

Sitting there in his exam room a wave of dread prompted a quick rush of tears. Something was telling me to have the surgery right away. The doctor agreed and scheduled it for that Monday, the day after Mother's Day. Because I was having so much pain, I wasn't even able to visit my mom, who gently accepted an apology for my absence, "It's all right Nancy. It's no big deal. I'll see you tomorrow when you go in for your surgery."

Dave and I arrived at the hospital around 6:30 a.m., an hour before the surgery. The bold character who had insisted on the ultrasound and then voted for the hysterectomy just three days earlier was in hiding that Monday morning. I heard myself informing the doctor that I didn't need the surgery after all. "If those people open me up and find nothing, they'll think, 'That lady's a big wimp!' And besides, I think the pain has subsided."

I woke up in the hospital room surrounded by loved ones. The doctor was at my bedside. He leaned down and told me they'd found a little cancer. There was that word, *cancer!* More bad news: the lab tests showed it had metastasized (spread beyond my ovary). But for some reason I was not reacting very strongly. Clearly I didn't comprehend what was really happening: my advanced stage of ovarian cancer could mean an end to my life!

My husband summoned his courage and broke the sad news to our teenage sons. Greg and Geoff could hardly believe what their father was telling them. They each reacted with denial and then, gradually, shock as the seriousness of my prognosis set in. Greg has since told us it was a surreal time for him and one that's still hard to talk about. We knew it had been rough on them, yet Dave and I agreed from the very beginning that we'd be open and honest with the boys and our family. There would be no toning down the truth to shelter them from the heavy reality cancer had dropped on our doorstep.

The Adventure Begins

The day before I was released from the hospital an oncologist came to my room to talk about the chemotherapy I would be getting. A nurse followed up with more details about what to expect, briefly explaining what I'd have to go through. My first response was, "Okay, but I work full-time. I'm not going to miss work!"

I felt the strong need to talk to my husband. I called him, crying on the phone. Next I called Sabra. She asked if I'd eaten any lunch and when I said no, she offered to bring something in. She showed up within minutes, spreading a little blue and white checked tablecloth out on my hospital bed. We had a bologna sandwich "picnic" surrounded with at least twenty floral arrangements sent by concerned friends and family members. Then Dave arrived. We talked. I felt calmer. With their help, I got through that awful day.

During my stay a man who'd been a patient at our physical therapy clinic stopped by to visit me. He said he was sorry to hear about my diagnosis, but that he felt I would be fine. "I want you to remember a word I've used for many years. It's 'salubrious'—I want you to *think* health. Salute each day with an image of healthfulness!" I was moved to think that this man would even remember me, much less visit me in the hospital.

He'd been a Medicare patient, and I'd merely escorted him from our clinic to his hospital appointment some time back, waiting for him to fill out his registration forms and so on. This gesture was nothing out of the ordinary for me as our clinic was located on the top floor of a same day surgery unit next-door to a hospital. To this day I remember "salubrious" and try to heed his advice.

Before I was discharged a vision came to me in a dream. In it I was standing in front of a group of people telling them how to fight cancer. The dream made it very apparent that my diagnosis would be the beginning of an adventure God had arranged for me. I couldn't resist the question, "Was the Dale Carnegie course part of the groundwork for His plan?"

That is how my personal journey with cancer began, in a hospital, under the cloudy verdict of my own humanness. It's a journey I've come to embrace as a blessing, a gift that's allowed me to reach others in the most intimate of settings—in the narrow space between hope and despair.

The First Round

"You'll need to buy a wig," my oncologist advised me in a lively conversation during my hospital stay.

I looked at him in shock, "Oh, I won't need a wig. My hair is really thick. It's not going to come out."

He pleaded, "Nancy, PLEASE go buy a wig."

But I wasn't convinced, "Are you *guaranteeing* my hair will fall out? I just don't think my hair will come out. It's very thick."

Life is full of ironies. I was proud that I'd finally grown my hair out to one even length just below my chin. To top it off, I'd had a perm about a month before surgery, achieving just the look I wanted. I was convinced I would not lose my hair, but the doctor was emphatic and gave me the name of a wig shop, telling me the owner would take good care of me.

In the privacy of my home I was forced to contemplate reality. I thought I was dying. It was that simple! I had cancer and I was dying. What can I do? I have a husband and two teenage sons. I can't die. I'm only thirty-nine! I'm too young. Resting on the couch, in the familiarity of my house, stark realizations destroyed any blurred vision of the future.

My three sisters and I sat and cried together. My minister came and prayed with me, asking God to give me the strength and courage I needed to fight the cancer. This is not some case of the flu, I thought. This is cancer. I must prepare for the journey.

Along with the mental preparation, I put myself on automatic pilot and darted around trying to complete a "before chemo" to-do list. Among the items on my checklist was what became a three-letter dirty word: "WIG." Next-door to a 7-Eleven and within burger-whiffing distance of a McDonald's, I found myself at the little salon my doctor had recommended, handing over $450 with my order for a hand-tied wig made of real hair.

The shopkeeper had shown my sister Carla and me an array of color swatches and tried to choose one that would match my own hair (which was frosted at the time). He measured my head. He pulled a little stocking thing over my scalp so I could try on different styles. It felt spooky, as if I were being outfitted with a prosthesis for a limb I still had.

I wasn't thrilled about the cost of the wig, but I followed doctor's orders. Imparting his wisdom on such matters, my doctor had told me I should have one of these "good" wigs, because I was a working professional. Offering this type of advice is probably as much a part of the oncologist's bedside manner as answering questions about chemo and diet, I thought.

My special-order wig wouldn't arrive for another five or six weeks (well after my hair was expected to wander off), so I headed to yet another salon to buy my interim wig. This little cheapo model was just $99, but overall, it ended up garnering more compliments than the good wig. Regardless of the price tags, the story we'd heard about our insurance company covering the cost of the wigs was a fairytale. Even after many phone calls and cajoling there was to be no reimbursement. We were told the cancer patient's wig is not a "permanent" prosthetic device and therefore is not covered.

⤎⤏

On June 1st I made my chemotherapy debut, launching the series of six treatments prescribed as follow-up to the surgery. I'd undergo one a month for the next half a year. I complained to the doctor that I couldn't start so soon, "My belly's not healed from the hysterectomy. The incision might burst open. Don't you get really sick with chemo?" At this point my stall tactics were useless, there was no delaying the inevitable.

Trying to be reassuring, Dave informed me that he'd spend the night at the hospital with me. I could see in his eyes how trying the last couple of weeks had been. It was difficult for him to be present for the treatment, but he wanted to help me through the first one.

I checked in at around 3:00 in the afternoon and was soon hooked up to receive I.V. fluids to ensure my body was properly hydrated for the chemo. I was told dinner would be coming in a while and afterward a nurse would start the "push" of Adriamycin and the Cytoxan I.V. The Adriamycin was in a jumbo-sized syringe with the diameter of a fifty-cent-piece. Sitting beside me on the bed, the nurse "pushed" the powerful drug into my arm at a slow rate to minimize the discomfort. Its sidekick, Cytoxan, hung overhead on an I.V. pole as I watched it drain drip by drip from a clear bag. At around midnight came the granddaddy of them all, a drug called Cisplatin.

I looked up to see the nurse remove the brown paper wrapper from the Cisplatin and hang the bag of fluid on the I.V. pole. She said she'd first give me a shot of Lasix to make me urinate more often—Cisplatin, a real bully in the chemo neighborhood, is so toxic it must be flushed from the kidneys as quickly as possible. With this in mind, I'd ordered a bedside commode and indeed, ended up spending most of the night on it. My body trembled every time I threw up and with each forceful emptying of my bladder or bowels. It seemed non-stop. With the I.V. in my arm it was difficult to maneuver—I had trouble even wiping myself. I had to ask someone to continually drain the vomit basin while a nurse kept emptying the commode.

I'd dimmed the lights of my room to bring as much calm to the scene as possible, but it was a futile effort. I shivered continuously. Dave and I heard the plastic tubing of my I.V. line rattle out an unnerving tune against the metal pole as I shook. To say the least it was not an easy night, but when dawn finally appeared I told myself, "At least you made it! If this is what it's going to take to survive, you can tolerate it."

By morning the doctor was in asking how I'd managed. I felt so drugged that I didn't know how to respond. Expecting the chemo to upset my stomach, he then prescribed a nausea-fighting drug called Ativan and said I should call him with any problems. "See you next week when you're in for your blood tests," he added with his casual farewell. Those tests examine both red and white cell counts to see how the body's tolerating the chemo.

I felt extremely weak. Dave had to dress me. Less than twenty-four hours after entering the hospital I was being discharged—*in a wheelchair!* I kept my head down as we rolled out. I knew many people in the hospital and was ashamed to have them see me in the chair, clinging to my little gold plastic puke basin. I didn't feel like seeing anyone that day! At home Dave got me ready for bed. It was about 9:30 in the morning. I slept until early afternoon, got up, and felt more or less okay. In what would become a post-chemo ritual, Mom and Dad arrived Sunday morning with donuts. Then my brother D.L. stopped in to say hello and have a donut. Thankfully, by then I could join them—at last I was able to eat something a bit more substantial than red Jell-O and tea.

I'd been warned that my hair would disappear in around eighteen to twenty-one days after the first chemo. The mutiny started slowly. I noticed that I'd begun to lose some hair but deluded myself into thinking it would just be thinning a little bit. I remember sitting on the couch, reaching my fingers up into my hair, coming out with handfuls, and methodically filling a nearby wastebasket. Dave asked me to please stop it, but I couldn't help myself. It felt like the hair was just hanging loose on my head and I removed it as instinctively as I would have brushed a loose thread from my clothing.

Taking a shower was a trial. As I shampooed, strands of hair would get stuck in tangles between my fingers. The thought of going bald made me cry. My son Geoff consoled me, "It's okay Mom. Your hair will grow back." He was still living at home and going to high school at the time. An eyewitness to the chemo and its aftermath, he saw (and heard) everything.

I decided I'd just get a haircut to deal with the balding problem. I called Sabra and asked her to cut it. There we were, playing barbershop on her back porch. She trimmed the remaining sparse hair so that it hung just below my ears. I thought the cut would work well until I absolutely had to wear the wig.

When she finished, Sabra put down the scissors and grabbed her leaf blower to chase the clipped hairs off of my neck. The blower was so powerful I thought she'd surely blast the remaining hair right from my scalp! I grabbed my head and yelled for her to turn the machine off before I lost ALL my hair. We laughed. I knew then and there, successfully thwarting the advances of a mad leaf blower, that having a sense of humor would be crucial to surviving cancer. It was also clear I'd definitely need to wear a wig in public; each glance in the mirror forced me to confront this uncomfortable reality.

My first day on the job as a wigged woman was a Monday. Feeling self-conscious, I *ran* from the elevator to my desk. Once there, my female co-workers assured me it looked "fine." "Oh. Wait a minute," said one of them, reaching up underneath the wig and tugging at a string. I was afraid it was the price tag, but it was just a long cord attached to the inside. With this brief interaction my "cancer comfort zone" had been established. These folks would be supportive; they were not going to gossip or point and stare. They became trusted teammates in my battle with cancer.

Another Helping

My second chemo treatment took place three weeks after the first one, on June 22nd. Like clockwork, in just twenty-one days the chemo had nearly bared my scalp, save for a few measly tufts near the front. Because they'd refused to jump ship, I sarcastically referred to these as my "loyal hairs."

Again I'd scheduled my treatment for a Friday, using Saturday and Sunday to recover my strength for work on Monday morning. My oldest sister Linda had just wrapped up another year of teaching grade school. She'd dismissed her class into the heaven of summer vacation and, turning in the other direction, drove from her home in Dayton, Ohio, to spend the weekend with me. I assured her it wasn't necessary for her to make the long trip, but being there to help out was her way of dealing with the cancer and I appreciated it.

My chemo routine went something like this: go home from work around noon, meet Dave at the house, change clothes and head to my doctor's office for blood tests before going to the hospital for treatment. After reading the lab results this time, the doctor had said my counts were too low to proceed with the second chemo, but I insisted, "I have to go now. I'm mentally prepared to go now."

He finally conceded, saying he'd decrease one of the doses to compensate for the low count. It was settled. My gut instinct to take charge over my own care was kicking in. The doctor called for a hospital room and reserved the only one available—a semi-private. Linda met me there later.

In the other bed was a chemo patient hooked up to an I.V. She happened to be a woman I knew. Her name was Janice, and she, too, had ovarian cancer. I noticed with curiosity that she was throwing up even though she'd not yet had her treatment. This was my introduction to "anticipatory vomiting," a condition that would later haunt *me* as well. The mere expectation of becoming sick actually makes one physically ill. Once the real thing hits, anti-nausea medication (which may or may not help) is available, but it carries various side effects. One such drug made me clench my jaws so tightly I could barely speak after I'd taken it.

My sister Carla came to the chemo session too, talking to me and staying by my side until midnight. She came over from work, having stopped on the way for carryout food, which she somehow managed to eat in spite of my retching. Sometimes I think we women are given a special capacity for functioning under bodily duress— whether we're dealing with our own sickness or caring for a loved one.

The next morning my co-worker stopped by the room. Mark had come from another floor of the hospital where his wife had just given birth to a baby boy. I was not wearing my wig. Only a few isolated strands of hair were hanging from my bare scalp. He stood at the foot of my bed telling me the happy news of his son's arrival, but his eyes were filled with a sadness I will never forget.

Linda chauffeured me home that day, where she became my cohort in a simple plot. Dave was out of the house. After my nap, the timing seemed perfect. We borrowed Dave's grooming clippers and headed for the deck out back. The sun bounced down the steep hillside and onto the rooftops in the valley below our neighborhood.

"There's not that much hair left," Linda observed.

"Go to it!" I directed.

In the beauty of that summer afternoon she clipped the remaining hairs until my head was nearly smooth. Along with Linda, I studied my new reflection in the glass door, not realizing Dave was on the other side.

"What are you doing?" my husband wanted to know, sliding the door open and staring. I looked at Linda. She looked at me.

"It was going to come off anyway. There were just a few strands left," I offered, but clearly it had upset him. Where was the resemblance to the girl in the wallet photo he'd carried since our high school graduation? It was surely not in the long blonde locks that curled in a perfect flip just past her shoulders...perhaps in the mischievous look in her eye?

Clean-shaven and renewed, I rejected the wig, found a lovely scarf instead, and tied it around my head in front of the bathroom mirror. There, that feels pretty good, I thought, and went back outdoors to bask in the warmth of a fading June day, my mind not far from the next treatment. I didn't know then how increasingly hard it would become to repeatedly undergo the chemo—a process that could save my life.

Anticipation

One of the most common shared nightmares we chemo patients endure is the extreme nausea and vomiting. Once you've gone through it with the first treatments, the apprehension over its impending wrath with subsequent doses becomes a mighty and powerful sensation. This fear evokes the "anticipatory vomiting" condition.

Even *thinking* of the chemo treatment would make me sick. Beyond that, the alcohol and Betadine I.V. prep, or just the sounds or smells of the place where it would be administered would make me distraught and bring about the gagging and heaving normally associated with getting the chemo itself.

In my case, the response was so strong, that as the elevator doors parted, revealing the big orange number "six"—marking the hospital floor where I would have the infusion—I'd begin to vomit. Dave would run down the hall to get a basin for me, but even smelling the plastic basin seemed to bring on more of the same reaction. The smell of the hospital gown nauseated me. So did the scent of the sheets and pillowcases, so I would try to remember to take my own linens with me.

One of the regular nurses, a woman named Rachel, always wore the same perfume. Fortunately, it was a gentle scent and didn't make me sick. My sense of smell had become so intense that I could tell when she was near, even while I was sedated and for years after I'd been her patient.

I knew that I had become so sensitized that something had to change or I'd never make it through the full course of treatments. On the advice of a friend, I decided to seek out the help of a psychologist. My health insurance covered the cost of the psychotherapy and I knew I had nothing to lose but the time I invested. The therapist tried to desensitize me to the experience. At our first session she began by asking me to close my eyes and enter a relaxed state.

"Feel the alcohol swab on your arm…it's okay…the smell of the alcohol is an odor that's okay." She guided me with the soothing melody of her instructions, "Feel the coolness of the Betadine… it's okay," and so on, until she'd mentally escorted me through an entire simulation of the I.V. prep.

In this state of relaxation I could sniff the alcohol and Betadine, and then feel them being applied to my arm without becoming ill. Both were used to clean the site where the I.V. needle would be inserted, and I'd come to associate them with the violent nausea brought on by the chemo itself.

I went to her for several sessions to learn a type of self-hypnosis. There were many rough times before I could successfully remove myself from the situation at hand. Before I learned the technique it had always felt as if the I.V. needles were being shoved about a foot up the inside of the vein in my arm. The poor nurses were just as afraid of me as I was of them. I'm sure they'd see me coming in for chemo and want to run the other way. It was always an ordeal for them to get the I.V. lines started.

Eventually, when I was able to focus extremely well, I could mentally detach from what my body was experiencing. The first time I was successful at this, Kimberly, the nurse inserting the I.V. that day, was completely amazed, "Oh my gosh, Nancy! The line is in and you didn't even know it!" She was right. I had no idea she'd just finished her task. I'd remained calm and nonreactive.

Unfortunately, as the chemo treatments continued, and worsened because of my growing intolerance of the medication itself, my negative response grew even stronger. Just going to the doctor's office to have the routine blood draw before the chemo sessions was enough to make me sick and fearful. By the time the big bag of chemo fluid was hung on the I.V. hook, where it would remain until every drop had drained into my veins, I was already vomiting, non-stop! These rough times took place before I started taking Zofran—a potent anti-nausea drug.

Given its potential to minimize the problem, I recommend the self-hypnosis therapy to other chemo patients. At least it provides an escape from what we all come to know as a horrible experience. I thought that I should be able to channel all that energy that was going into anticipatory vomiting—the negative interpretation—into something positive and useful. I asked myself, "If I can allow mere thoughts to bring about this strong, adverse physical reaction, can I flip the switch? Can I make thoughts work *for* me and reverse the growth of the cancer cells?"

I've been told that children going through chemo don't experience anticipatory vomiting. They just receive each treatment as if it was their first, not expecting anything particularly horrible to happen based on their previous encounter with the process. We adults, on the other hand, allow ourselves to become deeply programmed, to the point where the mere crinkling of the paper wrapper on the I.V. bag is enough to cause retching and heaving, despite medication to buffer the reaction!

Sisters' Weekend

"For there is no friend like a sister
In calm or stormy weather;
To cheer one on the tedious way,
To fetch one if one goes astray,
To lift one if one totters down,
To strengthen whilst one stands."

—Christina Rosetti, from Goblin Market, 1862

The third chemo session was in July and the fourth in August. What happened following the August treatment has become an infamous annual event. It is the unparalleled and shopping-riddled "Sisters' Weekend"—a time we four Satterfield girls celebrate the sisterhood we dearly cherish.

It began with a call from Judy, who lives in Cleveland, "I think it would be nice if the four of us got together. Carla could just drive across town, pick you up and head this way. Linda's coming up from Dayton."

I endured the regular Friday treatment, rested over the weekend and started back to work on Monday. I was feeling fairly tired, but just strong enough to plan for the trip at the end of the week. I telephoned Carla with a thumbs up. She was excited. "Great! I'll just pick you up from work and you can hop in the back seat of the car to rest. Don't worry," she said. This began a tradition of prized get-togethers, each documented by its own commemorative snapshot of the four of us.

The shot of the inaugural Sisters' Weekend gang shows me in the dreaded wig, which looks, to the untrained eye, much like a coonskin cap. Why didn't I just wear a baseball cap? I'd convinced myself that with the wig, no one would suspect I had cancer, never mind that my skin color was a frightening pasty white with a waxy sheen to boot.

We were quite the squadron of shoppers. No kids. No husbands. Just the four of us goofing off together. We started that first weekend with a trip to a Sam's Club on Saturday morning. What happened there probably would have sent most sane people home to bed, but the adventurer in me wouldn't hear of it.

In the spirit of Murphy's Law, we were somewhere near the *back* of the store when the sudden need for the bathroom yanked me to attention. I wasn't even sure what was happening, just that one of the precious little chemo side effects was kicking in. During my feeble attempt to rush to the ladies' room at the *front* of the store, Judy and Carla had to assist me, practically dragging my weakened body past the endless acres of merchandise. I was suffering a simultaneous onslaught of diarrhea and hot flashes. Both ovaries were now gone and my body reacted to the missing estrogen with sporadic heat waves.

The two of them kept asking from beyond the door of the stall, "Are you okay? Are you *sure* you're okay?" Once seated, I had taken off the wig and was using it as a makeshift fan.

I dabbed at my perspiring head with toilet paper, "Yeah, I'm alright. Just give me a minute." In fifteen or twenty minutes I put the wig back on and emerged from the stall for a quick check in the mirror to make sure it was positioned straight. We resumed our mission.

When we left Sam's Club I felt so tired I didn't think I could walk. I climbed in the back of Judy's van and stretched out for a short rest. "I think I could eat something," I told them. "Weird as it is, something fried sounds good. How about McDonald's?" And that was that. We pulled over for fries and, because the chemo really dried me out, a great big Coke. The combination seemed to sustain me.

We shopped all day, laughing and giggling our way through any store that caught our attention. Onlookers would have suspected we'd been drinking, but none of us had had a drop of alcohol. That night, tired and happy, we sorted through our heap of loot and agreed, this get-together must become an annual event!

In our snapshot from the following year I am wearing my own hair. It is only a quarter of an inch long, but it's mine. I am skinny as a rail, yet we sisters are together, still four in number, still spending the weekend fortune-hunting our way through craft stores and antique shops, making precious memories by the minute. In the years to come we'd target the outlet malls and Ohio's famous Yankee Peddler craft show.

Last year Judy drove her motor home to a state park and we four just hung out together. She gave us each a denim shirt with "Sisters' Weekend 2000" stenciled on it. One evening as we sat and talked she stitched a tiny flower on each one. Judy is "Miss Craft." She can make almost anything. She has even registered a copyright for the design for one of her stuffed teddy bears.

I am filled with gratitude when I think about the yearly weekend with my sisters. It's just one of the many gifts cancer has brought to my life; another is the frank realization that NOW is all we really have.

The Incredible Shrinking Wig

Another reason I hated wearing a wig, other than the fact that it looked terrible, is that it was sometimes too warm. My hot flashes, coupled with a particularly hot stretch of summer days, meant my scalp would perspire quite a bit. The result was a funky-smelling wig that made me feel like I was sitting in a gym locker.

I purchased special wig shampoo and conditioner to help keep the little mop looking perky and smelling clean. I'd wash it in the evening when I got home from work and leave it out on a towel to air-dry overnight. Not blow dry. Air dry. I took special care to follow all the instructions.

The first time I washed the wig I woke up in the middle of the night and checked on it, much as if it were a sleeping infant who might need his blankie adjusted. To my disappointment, the wig was still awfully wet. I replaced the towel with a fresh, dry one and went back to bed. In the morning the wig was *still* damp! What were my options at that point? It was tempting to give it a quick blast from the blow dryer but I resisted. My dilemma? I needed to get on my way to work and I didn't have time to wait for the thing to completely dry on its own. Reluctantly, I pulled it on and sensed the disconcerting feel of wearing a damp bathing suit. I "adjusted" the Velcro band and headed out the door.

Within just an hour or so of getting seated at my desk I felt a certain uncomfortable pinch. Why did the wig feel so tight all of a sudden? The drier the wig became, the tighter it felt, pinching my little crown in an elasticized vice. I began to have a terrible headache. It didn't matter that it smelled squeaky clean, how could I even *function* when the circulation to my head was being cut off?

Co-workers were starting to notice that something was wrong. I had to excuse myself to deal with the matter. Behind the closed door of the women's room I gave that wig a stern talking to. Taking it off and placing my hands on its opposite sides I assumed the archer's pose and stretched that sucker in every direction. Something had to give before the end of the workday, and knowing the laws of nature, it wasn't going to be the circumference of my head!

The wig became a sort of toy or prop for me. As my niece likes to remind me, at times I'd greet folks with a little slip of the wig just as someone else might tip his hat. "Top o' the mornin' to ya!" I'd grin. And if there are any advantages to wearing the wig, I have to admit, I did save money on hair products and costly salon services.

I developed a careless routine surrounding the wig, however. I'd arrive home from work in the evening, cruise down the driveway and hit the button for the garage door opener. At the same instant I'd automatically reach up and rip the wig from my head. Then, once inside the house and upstairs, I'd casually toss it aside like a piece of junk mail. On several mornings I could be seen frantically searching around the house for my wig, looking like those people who suffer from a chronic case of lost keys. "Geoff, Dave, have you guys seen my wig?" I'd shout in bullhorn fashion, eventually coming up with the lost goods.

Being the mother of a high school athlete is one thing. It has its own set of challenges...like how to politely disagree with an ill-advised coach or a ref who is clearly delusional. On top of that, for me, having cancer meant holding on to my wig at the crowded games, where there always seemed to be more fans than bleachers. I felt so self-conscious about the wig in the first place that the fear of it being knocked off stole my full attention from the game. This was especially true if Sabra was sitting next to me in the stands. She'd get so engrossed in the game that if such a thing existed, she probably could have drawn an "excessive jubilance" foul.

Embarrassing a kid with antiquated cheerleading skills is bad enough, but having his mom's wig end up at the free throw line could bring about a call of interference. It was a bit like that when I zipped down the highway in my convertible. I had to hang on tight. Would the state patrol write a littering ticket for a wig on the centerline? Could it be mistaken for road kill? I didn't chance it. Better to feel the wind through my hair than my hair through the wind!

One day Dave and I were at a stoplight in Wheeling on our way to one of Geoff's basketball games. In the car next to us was a little boy who I thought had stared at me just a bit too long. What choice did I have? I flashed him. My bald head, that is. I flipped the wig back off my bare scalp and watched his beady little eyes nearly pop out of his head. Dave was appalled that I'd use the old wig trick to frighten an innocent child. My defense? "The kid started it."

A Second Look

My fifth chemo treatment was in September. Football season had started. Dave and I are big sports fans, especially when it comes to West Virginia University, the hometown team. The year before, we'd had a blast in Arizona, cheering for WVU at the Fiesta Bowl. It was now fall and I wasn't going to let cancer keep me out of my usual spot in the stands at Mountaineer Field. My biggest fear was that someone would walk behind me in the crowded stadium and knock off my wig. Undaunted, we headed out to a game.

It seemed the summer heat had hung around a bit longer than normal and my illness had made me more sensitive to the sun. While the "Blue and Gold" zipped around on the field below, I was sweating my way through hot flashes. We had to leave long before the final numbers filled the scoreboard. It would be the only game I saw in fall '89.

A few weeks after that game I returned to the stadium but not as a spectator. Along with a few co-workers, I was taking part in the University City Classic, a two-mile fun run/walk. The football field served as the finish line. I was so jazzed up at the start of the race, that when I heard the gun, I took off like a bolt, racing down the first few yards of the course. Then I remembered I'd planned to *walk* the two miles.

One hand held my abdomen, still tender from the vomiting and the hysterectomy incision, and the other gripped my wig. It was a hot, difficult course, even though it wound around one of Morgantown's rare specimens of relatively level terrain. In my condition, it might just as well have been a sprint up Spruce Knob, the highest point in West Virginia. Still, I was determined to finish. I wanted the token ribbon and one of the Fun Run's souvenir plastic water bottles bearing the University logo, if for no other reason than to *prove* I'd finished. And not quitting is important!

I am reminded of this fact when I recall a particular day when Dave and I were leaving my parents' place after a visit. Sometimes the emotional pain of dealing with the cancer is almost as bad as the physical. At the end of our stay we said good-bye to Mom and Dad and headed out the door. Something made me start to cry. It was one of those times when the weight of it all—the cancer, the chemo, life— had pressed the last bit of composure from my shoulders.

I was already in the car when Dad realized that I was weeping. He charged down the driveway as the car backed out, scuttling along next to my window like a coach on the sidelines.

"You're not going to quit, are you Nancy?" he drilled me. "We Satterfields are not quitters, you know! Tell me you're not a quitter."

"I'm not a quitter, Dad," I reassured him, sniffling and thinking, okay, I guess I can run this play if I have to.

Eventually, after what seemed like a week in the desert, the Fun Run finish line was in sight. I'd made it to the football field in one piece, perspiring and practically gasping for breath. Along with several other participants, I dropped to the Astroturf for a rest. The wig had stretched with the warm sweat that covered my scalp. So much so, that when I tried to stand I was mortified to find that the hair had caught on the artificial turf, Velcro-like, nearly exposing my pale head as if it were a bright cue ball on a vast green billiard table! I quickly grabbed the wig and looked to make sure there were no witnesses.

⁂

The last of my six chemo sessions took place in October, the month of trick or treats. My oncologist had told me I'd need a CAT scan or M.R.I. when the chemo was finished, followed by a "second look" follow-up surgery. Despising the I.V.'s that accompany the CAT scans, I opted for the M.R.I. Compared to my recent adventures, it wasn't that bad—just an hour and a half of scanning my abdomen and pelvis for any sign of cancer. The result? An impressive "Clean and Clear."

Relieved, I readied myself for the second look surgery, planned for November. Thanksgiving was just around the corner. I looked forward to the whole family getting together. I always took special care to count my blessings on that particular holiday. I gladly envisioned telling everyone the good news of my clean bill of health. But that proclamation would have to wait. When it came time for the surgery, my red blood cell count was too low. I had to tank up on iron pills and move the surgery to the first week of December.

The twelfth month arrived, as aloof and chilly as it always is this far north. Entering the hospital, I felt strongly my medical adventure would soon be over. After the grueling chemo experience I welcomed the second look and thought of it as the final bend in the long, winding road I'd traveled since springtime. Just before surgery an O.R. doctor took a peek at my chart and remarked that my cholesterol was a bit high, not unusual in women who've had hysterectomies. "I can only fight one 'Big C' at a time doc!" I replied, knowing a little butter in my arteries would have to take a back seat to the more pressing concerns of the day.

Given my optimism, the news of more cancer hit me especially hard. Why hadn't the M.R.I. forewarned me? This time it was under my diaphragm. Just a few specks, but a few specks of cancer is not like a few specks of snow—the kind that floats down on these Appalachian mountains and disappears before you can reach for your hat. A few specks of cancer can change a woman's life, shorten it, or even end it.

It was this brutal reality embedded in the surgeon's discovery that made me ask him to step out of my hospital room. Then I lost it. I demanded an immediate appointment with God, "Why am I having to go through this? What have I done?" Instead, the knock at the door came from an I.V. therapy nurse.

"Nancy, do you want to talk?" she asked. "My name is Joyce. I'd like to say a prayer for you." She held my hand and prayed. As we talked I became calmer. I felt she'd been sent to me. In the ache of those few moments our friendship was born.

On the day of my discharge, waiting in my hospital room, wig situated on the summit of my cancerous little body, I was eager and ready to go home when the familiar heat of a hot flash rose in me. I grabbed the wig and tossed it against the foot of my bed. Just as I was tying my turban around my head, my minister entered the room.

"Yikes!" he said, nodding at the hairdo on the blanket. "For a second I thought you were lying upside down in bed."

We laughed. Then I told him I was going home, but that I wasn't clean. We prayed and talked a bit. A balding man, he joked that he probably had more hair than me. I argued, pulling the turban off to display some peach fuzz that had grown back despite my ongoing chemo. It was enough hair to win the bet and I reveled in my victory.

"I don't know how you do it Nancy," he remarked, referring to the bit of spunk I was able to muster under the circumstances.

I see it as putting on my game face. What real choice is there? When you have cancer, you have to play an active role in what is happening to you. I did it every day. It's not as if I never cried or got depressed. I did. I just waited until I was alone, usually after work, in my car.

At the office I was not a cancer patient. Only at home did I allow myself to have cancer. I'd hold in the emotion all day long, choosing to focus intently on whatever was happening at work. Then, during my short commute home, in the security and solitude of my vehicle, I could purge some of the sadness that weighed on me like rain-soaked clothes. A glance in the rearview mirror might reflect the fear I felt, my glistening eyes and tear-streaked face, and without fail, that awful, stupid-looking wig.

Taking It on the Road

In mid-December, just a couple of weeks after the second look, I met with my local oncologist. "I want you to go to Johns Hopkins," he said.

I was skeptical, "Why? Is something wrong? Haven't you told me everything?"

He sighed, and pointed at me with his ink pen, "Nancy, we're talking about cancer no bigger than the tip of this pen...grains of sand. I just want to make sure we're doing the right thing for you. I want you to see the chief oncologist there."

I agreed to his recommendation and scheduled a visit for January when I thought I'd feel up to traveling the nearly four hours to Baltimore. A tiny cynic inside was nudging me, "He's sending you over there so the *other* doctor can break the news that you're dying!"

One week into the New Year, in January of 1990, I found myself in a consultation room at Johns Hopkins Hospital, face-to-face with the chief oncologist. He began our meeting by saying he had read over the medical notes and seen the pathology reports sent from Morgantown. "I hate to tell you this, but I've concluded your cancer is at *stage four.*"

I shot back, "I don't care what stage I'm at, get me out of this mess! I want to be okay. I'll do whatever it takes!" For some reason, at that point of impact, when my ears first heard him indicate the situation was even more serious than we'd thought, I did not react with shock or surprise. It was only later I remembered that stage four ovarian cancer carried a life expectancy of just eighteen to twenty-four months! I wanted to have some input into my "life expectancy!" I was determined not to let statistics dictate my fate.

During that consultation Dave and I asked questions we'd written out ahead of time. I took a journal so we could make notes. The oncologist confirmed we were headed down the right path of treatment back in Morgantown, but my jaw dropped when he said the chemo dosage would have to be doubled for three to four treatments, "You can't do that! It will kill me! They make me so sick, I don't think I could manage it."

The doctor reassured me, "True, you will be a lot sicker than with the first six treatments, but you can handle it. If your blood count indicates you need a transfusion, you'll get one." He told me

I should definitely plan to stay an extra day in the hospital following the chemo because I could use the hydration. It was important to stay on schedule and get the treatments each month.

As he sat there fielding our questions, a gentleman knocked at the door, stuck his head in, and said he'd be in his office if anyone needed him. Instead, the doctor asked him to join us, and introduced the man as a gynecological oncologist. He introduced me as "...this lady from West Virginia who's had six courses of chemo and is *still* not clean!"

After a bit of discussion he asked, "Now, are you a physician? No? Then how do you know all of these medical terms?" I explained that I wasn't about to face cancer without knowing what was happening to me or to remain uneducated about what I was expected to deal with. He asked to examine me. I agreed and was told to step into the adjacent exam room. I unbuttoned the pearl buttons on my white mohair sweater. In fact, I was so nervous that I started to strip down completely until a nurse reminded me it was just a pelvic exam.

When he entered the room his eyes focused on my head. "Oh my goodness, you've got some hair!" he remarked. Only then was I aware I'd even taken off the wig!

He noted that I was healing well from the second look surgery and wanted to talk to me about some options that might be available at Johns Hopkins that were not offered back in Morgantown. First, I'd need to suck it up and get through those doubled-up treatments, which I hoped I could negotiate from four down to three. He told me to stay in the hospital an extra day for the vomiting and dehydration, and to take the transfusions if needed.

I didn't realize then as much as I do now, that what began as a simple knock on a door would be a crucial part of God's plan for my duel with cancer. This man would serve as a trusted physician, skillfully guiding my care for the next five years. I firmly believe that without his guidance and direction I would not be alive today.

The Double Whammies

A week after the trip to Johns Hopkins I started the double dose chemo treatments. My big concern was that I wanted to keep working full-time. "I've got to go to work!" I kept repeating to myself. The familiar routine helped keep me on track. The doctors told me I could still work, but that I would probably be off "a little longer than usual." What an understatement!

The double dose made me violently ill for the duration of my two-day hospital stay, then I came home full of anti-nausea drugs. Their side effects made it impossible for me to lie still for even ten minutes at a time. I was constantly in motion—always up and down—arms and legs continuously moving. I could barely stand it. I referred to the reaction as "scissors legs."

My parents would spend the first day at home with me. Their presence was reassuring to Dave, who worried about me while he was at work. I was extremely weak. After the first of those stepped-up chemos—I called them the "double whammies"—I knew how severe my reaction was going to be, making it especially difficult to plan the next treatment. There is no nice way to phrase it. They were absolutely horrible! Each time it took every ounce of my strength to re-enter the hospital.

I prayed that God would give me the power to get through them. I was always looking to the calendar for incentives, "Let me live to see Greg graduate from college. Let me be there when Geoff finishes high school! I want to be around long enough for this, survive to see that..."

The boys knew I was upset. Geoff gave me his hugs and reassurances in person, but Greg, who was in college and living on his own, would pop in for visits and scrawl short messages on grocery lists and memo pads for me to find later. These little notes of encouragement were often tucked in the overnight bag I packed for my trips to the hospital. They said things like,

Don't worry Mom!
You're going to be just fine.
I love you, Greg

and...

Mom,
Good Luck with your chemo treatment tomorrow.
You can do it!
Love, Greg

Knowing how hard it can be for boys to show emotion, their gestures meant the world to me.

My sons had a difficult time verbalizing their thoughts, and because I was fighting for my life, I couldn't give the maternal support that came naturally in other situations. We knew that the intense memories surrounding the loss of their eighteen-year-old cousin Ben in 1985, and the next year learning that their grandmother, Dave's mom, had cancer, only heightened their anxiety about my health. Picturing their cousin on his deathbed and imagining the same scene with their mother must have been frightening.

❧

Ben had struggled with neuroblastoma, one of the most common types of tumors found in children. For five years, from age thirteen to eighteen, this brave boy fought a tough but losing battle. When he knew the end was near, he told his mother (Dave's sister, Bette) that he wanted to leave their Virginia home for a few days and see this state one last time. He was born in West Virginia and had asked to be buried here, but first he wanted to scan the jagged green horizon again and once more travel the curving highway that led to his grandmother's.

I can still picture him during that last visit, standing in the sunshine with my sons, trying to take part in a simple game of whiffle ball. There were tubes leading from his kidneys and out of his back. The photos show his frail little frame looking especially vulnerable against a backdrop of West Virginia's immense hills. Still, Ben was happy to see Dave's mom, his beloved "Nana," and to breathe the fresh air at her country home, surrounded by the love and compassion of his extended family.

Just two weeks before he passed away, Bette called to say that Ben's time was near and we should come to say good-bye. I think it hit Greg the hardest because they were closest in age with just a couple years between their birthdays. Bette had warned us that her son did not want sympathy and that it might upset Ben to see his cousins shedding tears for him. Bette herself was amazingly strong during the loss of this very special young man.

When we arrived at the hospital I gave my sons some simple instructions before we neared his room. "You know how Ben is. He's trying to be strong for us, so we have to be strong for him. It's important to try and be positive when we see him. If you feel like you're going to start crying, just excuse yourself for a moment and step out of the room."

Because Ben had spent so much time at the hospital, he was a favorite patient of the nurses and doctors. One of the privileges he enjoyed was having a large, semi-private room all to himself. When we walked in, the curtain that divided the two beds was drawn. I'll never forget the shattered look on Greg's face when he pulled back the curtain and saw his cousin.

Ben looked as though part of him had already left us. His face was so thin. It appeared triangular in shape. He was bare-chested and tubes grew from his body like strings from a puppet. There were I.V. pumps and lines everywhere. The complicated machinery and his grave condition gave the place an ambience of surrealism. He seemed as knowledgeable about the life-sustaining gear as any medical technician. He knew what every beep and blip meant and monitored the equipment as carefully as a pilot checking the instruments while flying in a storm.

Living with a terminal illness myself, I now have a keen recollection of how Ben's attention shifted methodically from one person to the next that day, until he'd made his way around the entire room. His questions were directed at individuals, holding their attention in a succession of intense one-on-one exchanges.

"Have you been fishing lately Greg?" he'd ask, studying Greg's eyes and mentally tracing every crease of his smile.

"So Geoff, what sports will you be playing this year?" he continued, surveying my younger son's appearance with exactitude, then moving on to the next visitor in a calculated motion, the way a painter covers an entire canvas, a single brushstroke at a time.

I believe Ben was memorizing our expressions and studying the intricate details of our faces for what he knew would be the last time. In an eerie sense, it was as if he might need specifics to identify us at some distant point in the future and after a long separation had placed the rest of us in old age.

Sweet Ben died within a week of our visit. It was late July. We were on our family vacation at Nags Head, North Carolina. Our days on the beach had been stalled by rainy weather. Then, on the same day the sun appeared and put a bright sparkle in the tide, the phone call came. Bette gave us word that he was gone. Greg and Geoff packed up the beach chairs and their swimsuits. Dave got behind the wheel and the four of us made the sad drive back to Morgantown to bid Ben one last farewell.

⨍

My second double whammy was in February, on Dave's 40th birthday. I was discharged a couple days later on mine. Sabra tried to boost my spirits, "Have this chemo. Go ahead and puke your way through your 40th so you can have a lot more birthdays." The typical ruckus that goes with turning "the big four-O" and becoming "over the hill" could not have seemed more trivial to me.

As the hour approached for my treatment, the fear welled up in me. I called my friend Julie, frantically telling her I just couldn't do the chemo. She tried to settle my anxiety and kindly arranged to meet me at the doctor's office and then stayed with me at the hospital. I took so many pills to calm down that I couldn't remember going through registration. I desperately wanted the treatments to be over.

Later on, after I started to recuperate from the chemo, Carla hosted a small family birthday party for me at her house. I felt good being surrounded by loved ones and comfortable enough to go without the wig, as I now did routinely in my own home. The freedom to feel the breeze on my uncovered head was absolutely wonderful!

As one who'd spent her childhood days often in tomboy mode—fishing and camping with her brother and sisters in the West Virginia countryside—the chemo heightened my attention to hairstyle and appearance. In mid-March I phoned my neighbor to say I was ditching the wig. To celebrate we headed straight to the mall and bought some big earrings. But that wasn't the end of my celebration.

Harner Chapel has been our church for more than thirty years. Its bright white siding and pretty steeple give it the sort of quaint look Norman Rockwell might have paused to admire. Week after week its red double doors usher in the small congregation that has become my church family. The size of the place lends itself to the sort of intimate exchanges not possible in larger churches packed with hundreds of people. As in any family, we know when one of us has been ill or lost a loved one or suffered a tragedy. But we also know how to celebrate. Birthdays. Anniversaries. The arrival of a new grandchild. A promotion.

In church that Sunday the minister asked if anyone had something to share. I'd been sitting on my hands during the previous announcements, and his invitation was my cue. I thanked my church family for their prayers. I said I was just grateful to be there in attendance, and oh, did I mention, a bit of zip-a-dee-doo-dah in my voice, "I've flipped my wig for good!" How gratifying to proclaim my little triumph to the very people who'd kindly referred to me in their talks with God.

The Third Strike

The last of the three treatments was in late March. My sister Carla stayed with me in the hospital. It was rough going as always, but as soon as I returned home, knowing the chemo was safely behind me,

I began to feel a bit settled. The next big hurdle wouldn't come until May when my new doctor would perform another surgery, a "third look" to check for any remaining cancer.

In the meantime a problem emerged when I couldn't seem to recover from that final double whammy treatment. I grew weaker by the day and was always sick. There was no rebounding this time. When I'd get up in the middle of the night for a glass of water, I'd pass out. Dave would find me in a little heap and carry me back to bed. I can still remember the many times I woke up on the kitchen floor, my pajamas wet with spilled water. Dave didn't want me to be alone. He was afraid I'd pass out and hit my head, so friends took turns staying with me during the day.

Then things got worse. Eventually I couldn't even walk without passing out. My determination to fight this enemy forced me to *crawl* through the house when I couldn't stand. In my mind the formula was: stop moving and die! Creeping along, inches above the floor, from point A to point B, I focused on just one goal: survival. At times I could only move a few feet forward before having to stop and rest.

I couldn't keep anything down—not protein drinks or puddings, not even the recommended glucose water. I nibbled on Popsicles and sipped ginger ale. My neighbor Linda Anderson came over announcing she would cook for me. She thought the smell of something hearty wafting from my own oven would surely do the trick. She cooked her famous chicken potpie and brought me a small sample on a saucer. I fanned it a bit to cool it down and then took a bite. Dave saw me and was delighted, "Look! She's eating."

But by the time he'd left the room, I knew the spoonful wasn't about to stay down.

When I got to the bathroom I vomited violently. Linda was right there with me. Standing behind me, her caring arms wrapped tightly around my waist, she tried to support my body as energy drained away from me with every forceful heave. How could a little taste of home cookin' bring about such a drastic reaction?

Since the cancer, my overall appetite and my ability to eat certain foods and not others have rarely made sense. One time

Mom and Dad were driving me home from the hospital when I started feeling hungry.

"What sounds good?" my dad asked.

"Would you mind heading over to Kentucky Fried Chicken? I could go for some nuggets." My parents watched in a state of disbelief as I gobbled down the nuggets, coleslaw and fries. Every last disgusting morsel!

A similar craving came over me one day as Dave and I were driving to one of Geoff's high school games. "There's a Long John Silver's, Dave!" I said, ordering him to quickly pull over—as if I'd just spotted a shoe sale! In minutes I'd devised a makeshift dinner table out of the glove compartment and was woofing down an order of fish in all its deep-fried glory. He was worried about me getting sick, but I couldn't be concerned with such matters; I was too busy scooping up the little fried crispies from the corners of the empty box. What would my nurses say? (They'd warned me to avoid anything greasy or spicy in my diet.)

Linda's a medical professional and never got too excited if I got sick while she was visiting from next door. Sometimes she'd even hold the basin for me! She's a rational woman who always tries to be practical and positive. She was convinced my electrolytes were screwed up, to the point she was ready to draw blood and have it tested.

I was in a terrible predicament. I continued to call the doctor's office telling them about the situation, "I'm still throwing up—I can't seem to shake it this time." I was assured that as long as I was still going to the bathroom, some nourishment must be getting through.

One Friday Dave lifted me into the shower, bathed me, and set me on the bathroom floor so he could step back under the water to rinse off. "Don't move! I'll be right out to finish up and get you tucked into bed," he said. I dried off and crawled back to bed, not comprehending his instructions. Finally, he'd had enough. "I can't take this any more. That's it! I'm driving you to the hospital," he said, dialing the number to my doctor's office.

"I'm taking Nancy to the emergency room. She is not responding. She's curled up like a little baby. Something's very wrong!" he said, telling the person at the other end of the phone that this had been going on for two weeks. "She can't even walk." He was told to take me to the office, not to the hospital. They would have a wheelchair waiting for me at the rear of the building. Dave hoisted me up and piggybacked me down the stairs to the garage, where he set me in the car and gently looped the seat-belt around my emaciated body.

"Oh my God! How long have you been like this?" the doctor asked in shock when he caught sight of me. I know I must have looked pretty bad when Dave wheeled me in. I had a little bit of hair at the time but it was sticking out all over. My lips were cracked and my tongue was swollen from all the throwing up and subsequent dehydration.

"I'm going to take your blood pressure. Don't get up!" he ordered. As he suspected, it was extremely low. "Get her to the hospital! Go right to sixth floor, don't bother registering. I'll call to reserve a room." I began to cry, offering to eat lots of bananas to boost my potassium if it would keep me out of the hospital. "You could eat a whole room full of bananas at this point and it wouldn't help you," he replied. We drove off to the hospital in a rush where Dave quickly wheeled me right through the front doors to the elevators and up six floors.

When the doors parted and I saw the big number "6" and the territory made familiar by the rounds of chemo, the anticipatory vomiting began in earnest. The nurses were waiting for me in the room. Dave asked, "Are you going to stay with her? Someone needs to be with her while I go downstairs to get her registered." He was assured they would be.

"Don't worry," a nurse named Henrietta told him as they tried (and failed) to get an I.V. in me. For the most part the veins had collapsed, making the process especially difficult. Someone from I.V. therapy arrived and finally got it going, inserting the needle in the crook of my elbow, which forced me to keep my arm in a constant, straight position.

By this time the results of the blood sample drawn at the doctor's office were in. "Get her on step-down!" he commanded, "Get a heart monitor on her!" He knew my potassium and magnesium were critically low and there was no time to waste in helping me.

When Dave returned to the sixth floor room and couldn't find me, he was alarmed at first. No one seemed to know the nurse had taken me to the fourth floor where I was being hooked up to still more I.V.'s and having electrodes slapped on my chest. Two huge, quick-flowing bags of potassium were emptying into me—a very painful process. The pain was so intense one of the bags had to be taken off and my shoulder packed in ice for relief.

A nurse brought me a dose of oral potassium—pills so large even a horse would struggle with them—Dave got upset. "She's been throwing up for two weeks and you want her to swallow *those*?" He was just trying to protect me, "She can't take it!" But I knew I had to get them in my system and I did.

I thought, I must be dying! I recognized everyone standing around my bed but didn't know what was happening. My younger son Geoff had joined us and was trying to feed me ice chips. When they made it to my mouth I could speak for a bit. I was still throwing up—the I.V. bags were a powerful associative link to the dreaded chemo sessions.

By Saturday morning I was sitting up in bed. "What's going on? Why is everybody all worked up?" I asked. I was totally rehydrated and feeling back to normal, even able to eat. On Sunday I was so hungry I bribed Dave into bringing me some food, which I kept hidden under the blankets. I would graciously accept my meal tray bearing Jell-O and bouillon, and then privately tear into my secret stash. When the doctor stopped by that afternoon I begged him for a menu of solid food.

"I'm starving to death!" I pleaded.

"You can't have anything but liquids yet. You're just not ready."

When I confessed to the smuggling operation he changed my orders to a regular diet. During my discharge on Monday I even felt perky enough to joke with him, "You know Doc, I just had a case of P.M.S."

He was baffled, "What do you mean? You've had a hysterectomy."

I grinned, "Potassium Magnesium Shortage."

My comeback puzzled the staff. When I was admitted my level had been measured at 2.0, a far cry from the 3.5 to 5.0 considered normal. My heart was ready to quit. One nurse told me later on they didn't think I'd make it, "We've seen a lot. The odds were certainly stacked against you—we were afraid you'd never pull through." Imagine what their reaction would've been to know I was back at work on Tuesday!

As planned, I returned to the doctor's office later that week for a blood test because my hemoglobin had been low during the hospital ordeal. "You need a transfusion," I was told.

I flatly refused. It was 1990. There was still much concern about AIDS and the blood supply. "I've already got cancer, I can't handle anything else on top of this," I explained, offering to stuff myself with iron pills.

A nurse knelt beside my chair and probed gently, "Nancy, how are you feeling?" I admitted to feeling a bit tired. "Is your chest hurting?" she continued sweetly, as if she were going to break the news about Santa Claus.

"A little bit," I conceded, "I'm a touch short of breath."

"You're not working...are you?" she quizzed.

"Yeah. As a matter of fact, I just came from work."

She'd read the test results. In minutes I learned my hemoglobin was around 7.8—transfusion is usually necessary once it drops to 8.0. Still, I refused, "Sorry, I will not have any blood, thank you." Uncharacteristically, I promised to go straight home and precisely follow the doctor's orders. "I'll do whatever he tells me to do," I bargained. I went home, stayed in bed and took my iron tablets religiously. Luckily, I had another rebound in me and the numbers looked good next time around. Everything had to be in place for my next surgery, the third look, scheduled for May at Johns Hopkins.

CHAPTER 2

Miracles Happen

1990 - 1992

An Unlikely House Call

While I was still home recovering from my "P.M.S." nightmare I experienced a phenomenon I don't yet understand and have not shared with many people until now.

It was late in the evening. I'd said good night to Dave, who was tired and wanted to go to bed. I stayed up to watch an N.C.A.A. Final Four play-off being televised from Colorado. John and Sabra were attending the game, so between the free throws and lay-ups, I scanned the crowd shots looking for them. I thought maybe the network cameraman would catch Sabra leaping up from her seat to cheer for her favorite player.

After watching TV for a while I finally felt I should get some rest, even though I couldn't sleep once I was in bed. At some point I began to doze off. That's when it happened. I awoke to a flutter of small wings near my face and surrounding my head. What? What's going on? I blinked my eyes several times to make sure I was, indeed, AWAKE.

All around me were what appeared to be tiny angels! I couldn't make out their facial features, which were indistinct, but knew only that they *had* faces...and wings...very *busy* wings, which I both felt and heard! These little angels, about the size of doves, had no halos and were not brilliant white as often depicted in art, but instead they were a creamy ivory color. I felt surrounded by their warm energy and clearly interpreted their dance to mean, "Everything's going to be all right!"

Even so, I was completely frightened by the strangeness of the event. I got out of bed and went to the den to calm down. I wasn't dreaming. I wasn't on pain medication or any medication at all that would cause me to hallucinate. There was simply no way to explain this unlikely house call in any ordinary terms.

In my state of bewilderment I decided to phone my friend Debbie, who always stayed up late. She was a good friend of ours and had helped us out in so many ways during my illness. I was crying at this point and found it hard to describe the event. She tried to calm me down, "God's just trying to tell you everything will be okay." I forced myself to accept her words and returned to bed where Dave was still sound asleep.

This is between God and me, I repeated to myself. I had no physical proof of the mystifying encounter and no worldly explanation for it. I told no one over the next day or so. I'd been thinking a lot about the visit from those tiny angels when I decided to share my story with Denise, a woman at work. I respected her strong religious faith and appreciated the fact that she'd always been a comfort to me when I needed it.

Misplaced as it seemed, her first question to me was, "What *time* did this happen, Nancy?" When I told her, she got a shiver of goose bumps. "That's when I was praying for you! I was praying so hard that God would give you a sign," she said, reminding me to have faith in God, no matter what he might be planning for me. Since then I've made a special effort to do just that. After sharing my experience with Denise I felt free to tell Dave. I'd been afraid that, for some reason, he wouldn't understand, or that he might doubt what had actually transpired. I was wrong. He listened. He believed me. He wasn't even hurt that I hadn't told him right away.

The Correct Answer:
None of the Above

a) *shark cartilage*
b) *aloe cocktail*
c) *veggie delight*
d) *India goop and vitamins*
e) *none of the above*

If you ask me which alternative approaches have helped fight off my cancer, the correct answer would be "e) none of the above."

Imagine drinking an expensive, terrible tasting drink made from powdered shark cartilage and juice. I called it my "shark shake" and drank it with the "what could it hurt?" approval of one of my doctors. It had a terrible taste and left a disgusting chalky residue in my mouth that would stay with me the whole day. Besides tasting bad and costing lots of money, I didn't feel my shark shake was really helping me and ultimately ditched it for another supposed remedy.

Vegetarianism has its followers and for a brief while Dave and I were among them. We'd ventured to the local public library to hear a presentation about cancer and diet. Along with that topic we heard an inspiring appeal to adopt a vegetarian diet in the war on cancer. We decided it wouldn't hurt to give it a try in my "all-hands-on-deck" approach to surviving cancer.

We hired a vegetarian cook to prepare a week's worth of meals at a time. We'd pick up the food and have a seven-day supply at our disposal. We weren't always sure what we were eating, but we felt good. We'd just gotten the hang of it when she doubled her prices and the plan fell out of our price range.

Aloe is used in so many different applications that it made sense to me when I was told it could even help "eat away" cancer cells. With my doctor's blessing, I met with a scientist who'd developed a special formula. It was some combination of aloe and vitamins. As I understood it, the idea was to raise the pH level of the tumor so that it couldn't survive.

I was impressed by the apparent popularity of the treatment. While meeting at the scientist's office, various staff members interrupted our chat with questions pertaining to patients in several other countries, to an infant patient at U.C.L.A., and so on. It seemed to me everyone wanted in on the solution to cancer. I couldn't wait to test it out. Instead, in the most dramatic episode of my dabbling into alternative treatments, the aloe formula tested me!

After taking the prescribed half teaspoonful in a glass of orange juice, I became deathly ill. For seven days I couldn't stop vomiting. Along with that, I had a killer bout of diarrhea. At some point there was nothing left to empty from my bowels except a strange, yellow water—there was no stool to speak of! I spent twenty-four hours a day in bed, hooked up to an I.V., cared for by friends while Dave was at work (because I was too weak to manage the I.V. on my own).

After the first couple days of this little visit to hell, I placed a worried phone call to my Baltimore oncologist. He reassured me that I'd soon be fine. But in a few more days I developed a terrible pain in my abdomen. He became concerned that I'd suffered some sort of rupture and advised me to go to the hospital emergency room for an abdominal X-ray and a check of my electrolytes. Nothing showed up, but it was clear I should never attempt the aloe mixture again. In order to put back on some of the much-needed weight I'd dropped in the ordeal I was given the unlikely prescription of rum and Coke, "There are lots of sugary calories in it—drink up!"

My doctor had advised me to "Set parameters! If something's not working for you after three or four months, make a change." But in fact, other than a heavy-duty vitamin regimen and some supposed cancer-fighting goop from India, I didn't attempt any other alternatives that were too far off the beaten path.

If and when your very survival is hanging in the balance, you might be surprised at the straws you try to grasp. Looking back, I guess exploring the non-traditional approaches to fighting cancer was worthwhile. I came away with a reinforced belief that there simply are no silver bullets to kill this thing, even though my doctor had predicted the year 2000 would bring a magic cure for cancer.

But there's no magic. Recent history has shown not even a new millennium could deliver on such a challenge. For me, surviving has meant combining all sorts of elements, with no one approach holding the single key.

Living in the Woods

"The woods are lovely, dark, and deep,
but I have promises to keep,
and miles to go before I sleep..."
—Robert Frost

"If we find you clean, and I think we will, we'll surgically install a 'Tenckoff' catheter in your stomach," my Baltimore doctor was explaining just prior to my third look surgery in May. "When you wake up from the operation you'll feel a big bulky catheter tube which we'll use to administer your P-32, a radioactive isotope. It's a treatment that should zap any cancer cells that might be floating in your abdominal fluid. Hopefully, the P-32 will hold off a recurrence of the cancer."

This set my expectations in motion. I wanted more than anything to wake up in the recovery room and feel that catheter. Unfortunately, that experience would have to wait. The surgery had to be put on hold for a while when the pre-op X-rays showed something strange on the liver. The doctor sent me to radiology for an ultrasound, which confirmed the suspicious irregularity.

The doctor told me it could be more cancer, or maybe scarring from a bout with hepatitis, which could mean trouble handling the anesthesia. Now hours behind schedule for the surgery, he offered me the option of going home and returning in two weeks for a follow-up ultrasound before proceeding with our plans for the third look. I discussed the situation with Dave, my sister Judy, and Mom and Dad. I'd painstakingly prepped all night for this. My instincts said to go ahead with it. He'll open me up and see what's going on, I thought. It will be good to know where I sit. I gave him my decision and the doctor phoned the O.R. with the order to get ready for me.

In the waiting room my family anxiously anticipated word of my condition and received it one bit at a time, like the pages of a letter mailed in separate envelopes.

"So far so good."

"The biopsies look clean, even the liver. It was only some scarring."

"We think she's doing okay."

"We'll keep you posted."

My news came later as my fingers made their way over the multiple bandages strapped across my newly stitched midsection. I smiled groggily. It was there. I could feel it extending from my right side—the Tenckoff catheter. What a relief! I was enjoying this "post-op afterglow" when the surgeon came in to tell me that despite the Tenckoff, I was not, in fact, *totally* clean.

As he was closing me up, there, hiding in the nodes of my stomach lining, was a tiny troublemaker. His diligent eye had caught sight of one small, calcified tumor, which he promptly evicted. The next day I went to the radiology department and received the P-32, whose radioactive isotopes were on a "search-and-destroy" mission for any remaining cancer cells.

The drug looked simply like water in a bottle as it fed through the catheter and into the abdominal cavity. My body was rotated to complete the internal "washing." I was rolled onto my right hip, my left hip, both hips were raised, and then my head was lifted. I couldn't help thinking, that ought to do it, but I bet I'll probably need more chemo.

In the meantime I was feeling a bit like a nuclear power plant with a history of leaks. The staff that dealt with the P-32 suited up in the full regalia of hazardous material handlers. How could I not become just a tad apprehensive? My gut was full of a material so dangerous these folks didn't want to risk getting even a drop on their skin. When a technician came into my room to remove the catheter, I noted he too, was sporting the space suit look. I felt a little jerk of pain as he snipped my skin near the incision they'd made to install the catheter. He removed the spongy connection, placing the whole apparatus in a sealed container, and band-aiding my side with steri-strips.

A few days later I lay in my room recovering when the doctor came in, smiling. "The pathology is back. Everything looks clean," he said, and then made a wonderful pronouncement, "We consider you cancer-free!"

"There's no more cancer?" I asked, hearing the words as if someone across the room had spoken them to me. "What do I do now?"

Without pausing he replied, "Well, for one thing, there's no more chemo. You're done with chemo. Go live your life Nancy! Have fun. Do whatever you want to do."

His tone flattened, "Given that yours was stage four cancer, it will come back. I don't know if it will be in six weeks, six months or six years, but it *will* be back. You're always in the woods with ovarian cancer."

I pictured the beautiful tree-covered mountains near my home and recalled happy childhood days of camping in the woods. I didn't mind being in the woods. For now I was cancer-free. I could handle living in the woods.

Coming Home

Like a soldier returning home from a long battle, my adjustment to life without cancer took some time. After a year of chemo, medical appointments, hospital treatments, surgeries, and months of physical and psychological exhaustion, I found it difficult to recreate the existence I'd known before the "war." It was frightening to be cut loose from the routine that had redefined life for Dave and me.

Safe at home after the third look surgery in Baltimore and my doctor's words of warning, I broke down. For the whole year my concentration had been on the fight. I hadn't really grieved over the hysterectomy, the cancer itself, and all the other hardships. I could feel the tight seams I'd sewn around me give way, exposing a vulnerability that refused to be concealed any longer.

I looked around our home and thought how unfair it seemed that we'd moved in just a short two years before the cancer hit. Hardly time to get settled in. Hardly time to enjoy this beautiful, quiet neighborhood. We'd spent so many years in the previous house, raising our two sons from babyhood to their teen years, chasing back and forth from home to the ballpark and nearby playground. We were close to the ice skating rink and schools, even our church, during all those years when the four of us formed a small huddle of momentum that seemed to always be en route to something.

Depression set in during my recuperation, just two days after feeling relieved and grateful to be declared cancer-free. I'd been filled with happiness when we returned home from Maryland. I was welcomed by giant pink ribbons tied around the big maple tree in the front yard and the prayers and celebration of my friends.

Sabra had adopted the "shout it from the rooftops" approach to announcing my good news. She yelled out loud to total strangers in the bleachers at her son's baseball game, "Nancy's cancer-free! Isn't that great? Nancy's cancer-free! No more cancer!"

As for me, I'd made tons of phone calls from my hospital bed at Johns Hopkins, calling friends and family members, ignoring the long distance fees in favor of proclaiming to anyone and everyone, "It's over! I'm done with chemo! I'm cancer -freeeeeee!"

So why did I begin to feel so low? I called the doctor. "What's happening to me?" I asked.

"We were wondering when this would all catch up with you— you've shown such strength through this ordeal," I was told, and then offered medication. I declined it, and instead looked to time, prayers, and the support of friends to heal the pain and sadness I was feeling.

Eventually, a sense of normalcy returned, interrupted only by the powerful responses I had to my follow-up appointments, especially the first one. The association was emotional, and so strong that I'd become physically ill at the thought of returning to Baltimore and walking back into that hospital. In June, during the drive out for my six-week check-up, I was taking Ativan to fend off the nausea. The drug also acts as a sedative, which worried Dave, "Honey, you're going to have to quit taking those or you won't even be able to get out of the chair when they call you."

I kept saying, "I don't think I can do this." The overwhelming fear of reentering the hospital was born in the memory of my anxious days there, and the expectation that new cancer would be discovered and more chemo prescribed. I knew my tenuous future rested in the hands of my doctor who could, in the time it took to speak a few simple words, cast serious doubt on my chances for survival.

Dave pulled the car into the parking garage at Johns Hopkins. I immediately rolled down the window and vomited. He had to get a wheelchair to take me inside. Every few months I got another check-up under my belt, and medically speaking, they were all uneventful. Even so, there was always some apprehension lurking in the appointment book.

Losing Aggie

It's been said some people need permission to die. Others sense when the time is right for letting go and then release their grip on the reins that have held them in place, however precarious that hold might be. I've always believed this was the case with my mother-in-law Aggie.

She'd suffered for nearly four years with lung cancer. Within three months of getting word that I was cancer-free, she let go. I thought she'd held on, struggling, until the peace of mind that came with my clean bill of health allowed her the freedom to pass from this world and all its physical flaws.

Aggie was the kind of person who took it upon herself to look over those around her, especially anyone in need. I think she imagined herself resuming her grandmotherly role in the next life, joining her grandson Ben. He was her first grandchild and she'd sorrowfully watched cancer claim him just a few years before.

Although she'd been in remission, after my diagnosis, a recurrence set in. The two of us ended up taking chemo treatments together. We'd even had some of the same chemo drugs prescribed for us. I know what they did to me, and the drugs were even harder on her, a woman in her sixties. The mutual experience wove a special bond between us. It was easy to empathize with one another and understand what we were each going through. For more than a year Dave lovingly chauffeured his mom and me to treatments, week in, week out.

Aggie was an inspiration to me because she had fought so hard. In the end the cancer that had invaded her lungs, and the stress of chemo and radiation, weakened her body to the point where she could no longer endure the battle. As it happened, Aggie and long-term survival were not suited to each other. I attended her funeral, consumed by a powerful, stark sense of my own mortality and the strange singed taste of survivor's guilt fresh in my mouth.

Things That Go Bump

As a matter of routine I examined myself for any suspicious lumps and bumps that might have found a home—especially in my neck and under my arm, where I knew the doctors always looked. One day in December of 1991 I felt a little something in my groin. It seemed to be a small nodule. I dialed Baltimore and spoke with my doctor, "What do you think this is?"

He advised me to go see my Morgantown oncologist for an exam, "Then keep your mitts off it! Don't touch it for three days. If it's still there in three days, call me back."

I took the first part of his advice and saw the local doctor but I couldn't stop touching that little lump. When you know something's there that's not supposed to be there, and you're not sure what it is, curiosity takes over. My physician urged me to head to Baltimore and have it checked. There the second doctor felt the bump and immediately decided a biopsy was in order.

"Give me a twenty-gauge," he told the nurse.

"You're not gonna shoot me, are you doc?" I joked. When he inserted the large gauge needle and began to draw a pale gold liquid up into the syringe it was evident this was no time for wisecracks. I saw him make eye contact with the nurse and knew immediately what they were thinking…it's back…the cancer's back.

"I'll rush this through pathology and call you in the morning." Like the unexplained "bump in the night," his words echoed loudly in my head during the drive home to West Virginia. At work the next morning I reached for the ringing phone and heard his voice on the line.

"Nancy?"

I jumped in, "It's back, isn't it?"

"How did you know?" he asked. I told him it was the look on their faces that gave it away. "We'll do surgery and biopsy the nodes on either side of it to make sure it hasn't spread. Now, when do you want to have the surge—?"

I cut him off, "Yesterday!"

His surgery schedule was always booked, but I pressed him, "I want it now! I'll go as soon as you can get me in." His wife, an oncology nurse in the same clinic, phoned the next day to say there was an opening the following week. "I'll be there," I promised, and hung up the phone feeling like I'd just shook hands on a dicey deal.

It was 5:00 a.m. on December 16th, the day of my surgery, just days before the official start of winter. Mom, Dad, Carla, Dave and I drove into the winter sunrise, once again passing through the ancient mountains that form the Eastern Continental Divide. I noted the familiar sights along the way, inhaling the gray-blue beauty of the hills and knowing that, within hours, the sterile landscape of a Johns Hopkins operating room would be the next vista on this journey of mine.

The standard prep involved getting an I.V. started and then, assembly line fashion, making one's way to surgery and eventually, out to the recovery room. The line began in a big room with I.V. chains hanging from all over the ceiling. It could have been "Ladies' Night" at the surgical ward. It was filled with one apprehensive woman after another, seated in her hospital gown, loved one at her side, awaiting her surgery.

"I can't do that. Please don't make me do that," I begged, looking out into the big room. I knew the nausea would begin with even the simple Betadine prep of the insertion point and that the vomiting would start as soon as the needle slid into my arm.

"What's wrong?" my doctor asked.

"It's the association—it's just so strong. I can't go out there and puke in front of all those women," I pleaded.

The staff was very kind and let me wait on my own in a private room, "We'll keep you back here as long as possible. If you start having problems after we put the I.V. in, we'll give you something to help."

"Okay," I said, thankfully, "But have it right here, ready to inject, because I know I'll need it." And I did.

I woke up after surgery in recovery, sitting there with my surgery cap on sideways and trying mightily to get my bearings when I heard my doctor say, "Hey, have I ever shown you pictures of my kids?" He was telling me to down my crackers and ginger ale so he could let me head back home. I did as I was told, crunching and sipping as I gazed at snapshots of his offspring.

"We're putting you on a drug called Tamoxifen," he announced. "Your pathology slides—the estrogen receptor tests, E.R.T.'s—show traces of the hormone. This drug will act as a sort of anti-estrogen agent and should retard tumor growth. You're probably going to gain some weight and have a few hot flashes, but you'll be fine. I think this will work," he proclaimed confidently.

And with that, my entourage and I made the U-turn and headed back across the mountains. I lay on the back seat of my parents' van, contemplating the events of the day until we finally pulled onto our street at around 8:00 p.m. I remember having trouble walking. The incision in my groin was fresh and painful. I felt stiff from lying down during the entire trip home.

On the pavement in front of the house there's a little rise that I call our speed bump. I could not negotiate the speed bump that night—it was too painful to lift my foot over it as I walked. When I eventually made it inside I wanted only to sleep and was in bed by

9:00. If I were going to make it to work in the morning as planned, I needed my rest.

"Are you supposed to be here?" my co-workers asked the next day in disbelief.

"I'm fine," I assured them, "I just had this little node taken out. I'm okay, really." I checked my bandage during the day and found that it was draining (maybe because I wasn't to be up and about?). It was lucky for me that our office was in a medical building. I walked downstairs to the same day surgery office, "Can you folks re-bandage this incision?"

"When did you have surgery? Yesterday? Are you *supposed* to be at work?" they wanted to know.

"Oh, I don't know...no one really said not to. Besides, I make my own rules regarding these things." They fixed me up with a new bandage and I left work.

Just inside the door of my home, I heard the phone ringing and grabbed the receiver. It was Johns Hopkins. "Hello. This is the nurse at the surgery center," a voice greeted me from the other end. "We're just calling to make sure you're doing okay and not having any problems." I assured them I was fine, secretly relieved I'd been there to take the call and minimize their inquiry into my whereabouts.

Sure, I was sore for a while, but it wasn't bad. Christmas was coming in a matter of days. There were still cards to send and gifts to wrap, and then there'd be packages to open and treats to eat. 1991 was quickly drawing to a close. Brooding over a little cancer surgery was not on *my* to-do list. I believe God gave me the courage to keep looking forward and the strength to fulfill whatever mission he'd planned for me. Giving up or giving in simply would not do.

Sky's the Limit

If you're going to live life, have fun, and make the most of it, you need to get your priorities in order. For me, that meant making a list of the things I wanted to do and deciding which one I should attempt first. It was tough. I wanted to fly a plane. I wanted to parasail. The selection was endless. Skydiving seemed a natural first choice.

I wanted to do the things you can only do if you're willing to live on the edge. I wanted to tackle the stuff we all put off with mediocre excuses like, "I'll get to that when the kids are grown, when I'm older, when I have more time, when this happens, when that happens, when (fill in the blank)_____." For me, there was no more putting things off, no more "when." There was only "now!"

I enthusiastically recruited an ensemble of six friends and co-workers to join me. My future daughter-in-law Tricia and her mother were among them. Like me, none of them had ever jumped out of a plane, but we all agreed it sounded like fun. The others were mostly graduate assistants who worked with me at the clinic, including a young woman who was to be a bridesmaid in her sister's wedding the following weekend. Her mother had issued a strict warning, "If you break a leg or sprain your ankle before this wedding, I'll kill you!"

When the date arrived we made the trip to Summersville, about two hours south of Morgantown. The gang wouldn't let me make my jump first. Instead, I was forced to live through theirs. Dave, who was terrified, kept his feet planted firmly on the ground, and watched with me as one after another, they each made the plunge. I was thinking, okay, so far so good. No broken bones. Nothing out of the ordinary. I'm not afraid of heights.

These were tandem jumps, so the major responsibility rested with the professional skydiver who accompanied each of us. We were securely strapped to him in a harness apparatus. The excitement built all day long until it was my turn at around four in the afternoon. My comrades kept teasing me.

"Boy Nancy, what are the odds?"

"Hope yours opens!"

"How many times can this guy pack the chute and jump in one day?" The answer: at least once more.

I'll never forget the sheer exhilaration I felt, swimming through the sky, the thrill tickling every ounce of my being. Always in favor of documentation, I'd opted for the in-air videotape of my jump. I still like to watch it. There I am, peeking through my goggles and aiming a giant thumbs-up right at the camera.

When you've beaten cancer, what's a little plunge from 12,000 feet? I'd gained my weight back after dropping to nearly 100 pounds. My hair had grown in. I looked good. Felt good. It seemed life couldn't be better. The next day I spoke at a cancer survivors' luncheon. Still on a high, I whipped out my skydiving video and proudly illustrated how very much alive I felt!

Fasten Your Seat-Belts, It's Going to Be a Bumpy...

The sky is big. I was meant to explore it on more than one occasion. During a trip to the Bahamas I got a taste of parasailing. What a sense of freedom! I was elated to find myself kissing the breeze above the ocean. Scanning from the shore out to sea, I noted with awe the beautiful gradations of blue.

I waved gleefully at Dave and our friends on the beach, but wait, what were those stern looks they wore? Oh, just concern because they'd been told the day was much too windy for safe parasailing...and there I was, their favorite cancer survivor, whizzing overhead like a grape in a slingshot.

West Virginia has some of the world's finest whitewater rafting. It's a big part of the tourism industry in this state. Every year thousands of thrill-seekers venture onto the water and pound their way through the swirling rapids. Just two years after my hysterectomy and a year into being cancer-free, I was among them.

My boss John was given a pair of tickets for a rafting excursion as a thank you for a donation he'd made to a fundraiser. Those tickets made their way into the hands of two known adventure-seekers, my friend Julie and me. Not everyone in our raft was experienced with navigating the whitewater—in fact, only *one* of the six passengers had ever been rafting!

The Cheat River is a familiar landmark in this area. Through the eyes of the layman, it looks lazy and relaxed from a distance, but like a bobcat in a shallow sleep, in a flash it can put your agility, stamina, and survival instinct to the ultimate test.

On the day of the outing Julie and I showed up like sassy junior high kids ready to take over the playground. We boarded the raft with the others and headed down river with a tickle of delight in our bellies. We crashed through the first set of rapids laughing and exhilarated.

"Keep your paddles in the water!" the guide commanded furiously. But his words fell on the deaf ears of his novice rafters. The second set of rapids came upon us in a mighty rush. Another guy and I were tossed from the front of the raft and into the snarling white water.

My foot caught between some rocks, holding me hostage until I frantically freed it, leaving my tennis shoe wedged in the stone trap. The current sucked me along and under the raft, where I yelled between dunks, "HELP ME! HELP ME!" Terror rose in me until I popped to the surface and was scooped safely back inside. I made a clumsy beeline to the rear of the raft, my lone shoe squishing river water as I staggered. I shoved my foot under the butt of the biggest, tallest person in the raft, a man twice my size sitting right in front of me. There, I felt certain that *no* blast from the Cheat could joust me from my most secure mooring.

After we paddled to shore for our picnic lunch I examined my scrapes and bruises, briefly mourned the loss of my shoe, and openly admitted to my weary shipmates, "This is a riot! I'd go again if I could!"

The hot air ballooning trip was another fine adventure. It was part of the annual Mountaineer Balloon Festival that attracts balloonists and spectators from all over the country. I'd watched the colorful globes floating over these hills, as gracefully as the bright down from a milkweed pod. I wanna do that, I'd thought many times. So when opportunity knocked, I ascended.

The clinic had received a couple of complimentary ride tickets in connection with some radio advertising. But to whom should they go? Naturally, John and Sabra had first pick, but when John said he didn't care to go, his ticket found a home in my eager little grip.

It was really cold that autumn Saturday when Sabra and I, brimming with excitement and anticipation, headed out to the airport at 7:00 a.m. As luck would have it, the wind was too high or out of the wrong direction for the mass ascension that our balloon was supposed to be a part of. We dragged home like trick-or-treaters on a rainy Halloween. A second trip out met with the same conclusion. But the third time was truly a charm.

I love the memory of climbing into that basket, my breath stolen in the brilliant grace of the mass ascension. We rose slowly into the air and then floated in the space that seems a touch closer to heaven than earth. I was enamored with the peaceful silence of the trip, interrupted only by the burner whispering rhythmically into the "envelope" of the colossal dome. Because the balloon moves *with* the wind, there's no sense of being moved *by* the wind. Instead there's just the sense of being suspended in the blue, with a profound invitation to relax and dream.

As we descended we could see cars and their passengers driving along Route 705, the tops of trees and buildings, and eventually, home plate—that spot where our hot air adventure would end. In preparation for landing we were told to bend our knees because the basket would likely tip as it hit the ground. I was game. Any added bit of excitement tantalized me. But all too soon the flight was over, and without a hint of mishap.

Once on the ground we took part in a prescribed ballooning ritual. It involved sitting there on the grass, facing the sun, hands behind the back, and a glass of champagne positioned in front of you on the ground. The trick was to lean forward, pick up the champagne glass with your teeth and drink from it without spilling—a sort of tribute to the gods for a safe voyage.

Another challenge also took me to the air. I'd always wanted to fly a plane. Lucky for me, lessons were available in a nearby town and Curt, the instructor, was willing to take me on. Well, at least that's what he said before our first session.

I was giddy with excitement, but the man in charge had no time for giddiness. Curt didn't appreciate the fact that I brought along peanuts for our in-flight snack. He didn't think it was funny when I unhooked my dangly earrings to keep them from catching in the headset and was critical of the fact there was no glove compartment to store them in.

He wasn't amused when I asked if we could fly the little Cessna over my parents' house since we'd be so close to their home en route. My dad had said he'd be outdoors with his video camera just in case I came into view. Curt sternly explained that flying was no game and there was no time for airborne social calls, "There are lots of laws and regulations we need to follow," he said, leaving the scorched scent of a scolding in the cockpit.

"What if we pass someone we know?" I joked, "Is it okay to wave?" I persisted, pushing the poor guy to mile-high frustration, "Hey, does this thing say 'student flyer' on the back when you're out giving lessons?"

Now, when I look at the photo taken of me that day, standing near the plane with my one-shot instructor, I can understand his intolerance. What had possessed me to show up for this solemn occasion in flowered leggings and a ruffled, over-sized shirt?

Amelia Earhart, I was not! Still, when I took the controls for that brief brush with greatness, I could easily imagine the intrigue that had commanded her into flight. Soaring through the clouds with the little engine humming dutifully, the cares of the world below in a smear of green, I was more keenly aware than ever of the meaning behind my mantra: NOW really *is* all we have.

CHAPTER 3

Counting My Blessings

1994 - 1995

"Miss Ovarian Cancer 1989"

In a town built on a succession of hillsides, having a yard flat enough to support a vegetable garden puts one in a select but sparse crowd. So at the beginning of summer, when the little shoots that sprout in backyard gardens are stretching their fresh green limbs toward the sky, you can almost hear the shouts of joy. At the same time, I'm busy with a grateful little ritual of my own.

While the gardeners are busy weeding and watering, I can be found planning my ensemble and gearing up for my perennial lap at the Relay for Life. Each year this American Cancer Society fundraiser draws cancer survivors, their families and friends, and a crowd of well-wishers and supporters to the University track.

Those who take part in the Relay have asked sponsors for simple donations or to fund them, so much money for every lap, whether they walk or run. The initial lap, however, is strictly reserved for the folks who've been diagnosed with cancer.

The first year I was one of just nine (!) in the thin line-up of survivors. Sporting our Relay sweatshirts, we linked arms and bravely made our way around the track. It was a great night. We stayed until around midnight, hitting the track whenever we felt like it, and eating pizza to keep us going.

Another year we were given red sashes to wear. It was a nice gesture, but frankly, I found them to be a little plain. I made a quick trip to Wal-Mart and found the aisle where they stock those adhesive letters and numbers for mailboxes and signs. I picked the ones I needed to spell out my new self-proclaimed title, including the year of my diagnosis, "Miss Ovarian Cancer 1989."

Heck, I'd never been a queen of anything, why not elect myself? I got a lot of strange reactions the first time I walked down to the track. There were some mixed emotions, but mainly the effect I'd hoped to create, "Look at her! She's surviving ovarian cancer!" People asked whether I'd really been diagnosed in '89 and wondered how I'd managed to hold on for so long. I felt I could be an inspiration and offer hope to people who might be contemplating whether they, too, could beat the odds.

In following years I saw "Miss Breast Cancer" show up for a lap with the rest of the survivors. Others found their own good luck charms and little icons to decorate their sashes. It made me feel good to have started a trend that allowed people to show their individual pride in their participation. I still have my original sash. It's a bit tattered from so much wear, so I actually had to make a second one. I like having two to my name. One year I added a balloon hat for a touch more color. I take pride in my survivorship and in the little things that remind me of it!

Each year the event grows. There seem to be more survivors than the year before. We eye each other, taking a sort of human inventory as we line up for that first lap. It's always great to see so many people returning, but sad to know that some are missing and will never be back.

In the beginning, the idea was that someone from each "team" of walkers would be on the track at all times. As one person left the track for a break, another would simultaneously take off, relay-style. Back then a couple guys from work would come out and walk in support of me. It was a relatively low-key event. But in the last couple years the tailgating has become fairly extravagant and the entire event has grown beyond anyone's early predictions. This year there were more than 2,000 people in attendance.

For instance, on our team alone there are probably forty or more walkers, given family and friends, and the people who show up from work. The folks from the office make a big deal out of it. This year they contributed $5 to our United Way piggy bank to "dress down" at work that day, wearing their Relay for Life t-shirts. That night at the track we all gather under a big tent full of food and refreshments and make a company party out of it.

The feeling I experience each year at the Relay lifts my spirit. It's a poignant moment when I complete the lap with my cancer "teammates." It's as if we are each saying to the world, "There, I've done it. I've crossed the finish line in another year of surviving cancer." There is a sort of reverence that settles on the place while we make our way around, some of us weaker and more battle-weary than others. There are tears and hugs, smiles and congratulations.

The sight of all the survivors wearing their banners and marching en masse is truly stirring. In the most recent Relay they numbered more than 200, yours truly included. One of the survivors new to the 2001 line-up was my friend Carol Brautigam. For years Carol and her husband Jack had walked in support of me, but this year, just a few months before the Relay, she was diagnosed with breast cancer. This year, Carol walked *beside* me!

If ever you choose to see the personification of mortality and courage, the Relay is the place to be. There are survivors of all kinds of cancer. You'll see males, females, people of all ages and different faiths and racial backgrounds. Different languages can even be heard as the crowd moves along the track. There are survivors who look to be in their nineties. There are babies. This year there was a little two-year-old in a stroller, a bright survivor's banner wrapped around his tiny being.

There was also a woman who appeared to be quite elderly, with a painful-looking hump at the top of her back, gripping her walker as she made slow, sure laps. She was accompanied by a little boy of about five or six who was dressed in a bright red clown suit, his head shaved to a very short, "chemo" buzz. With his right hand on her walker and the left one carrying balloons, the pair rounded the track as routinely as they might have walked through the grocery store. For onlookers, I think the two helped illustrate the indiscriminate nature of this disease, and the perseverance it takes to keep battling, whether it's one mile or one footstep at a time.

At many of the Relays (they're always on a Friday night) I had just received my regular Friday afternoon chemo and couldn't stay for the whole evening. Sometimes I didn't even want to go, I felt so lousy. But Dave would get me fired up, "Okay Nancy. Let's get going!" And somehow the adrenalin I needed would take over, making me feel strong enough to get out there with my fellow survivors. I'd make that first lap with pride, shivering all the way, unable to keep myself warm in that icky post-chemo recovery state, and *then* I'd go back home, at least knowing I'd done it—one more time for the sake of saying to the world, "It's me, I'm still here, Miss Ovarian Cancer 1989!"

Taxol, Fireballs and Toasted Cheese

Five relatively calm years had passed since my hysterectomy and the first cancer diagnosis. I'd been on a steady protocol of Tamoxifen since the surgery to remove my groin tumor in December of '91. It was now May of 1994. My blood tests showed that the tumor marker, also known as a CA-125, was creeping higher. The marker (which is often used to monitor the elevated protein levels in ovarian cancer patients), along with pelvic and rectal exams and an assessment of how I look and feel, are all used to help pinpoint my status.

CAT scans also pointed to tumor progression. My oncologist, who was now practicing at Sinai Hospital of Baltimore, shared the inevitable, "We're going to have to do another surgery. I can palpate some tumor growth, and given that the marker's moving up, we better go in for a look." Just what I need, I thought, another huge scar on my belly!

He explained that this time they'd do what's called a "debulking." It's a process that involves taking as much of the solid mass of the tumor as possible, then scraping around it to get any straggler cells. I assumed I would be getting another chemo after the June surgery, given that the Tamoxifen had "fallen asleep on the job," allowing the cancer to progress.

While preparing for the operation I warned everyone at the hospital about my adverse reaction to starting the I.V., sharing my distressing history of sudden-onset nausea. They were all so kind. An especially nice doctor spoke to me as he gently inserted the needle into my arm. He had the magic touch—there was no vomiting! This was a first in the Nancy Chronicles of Surgery Prep.

Just before the procedure, several medical residents came in saying they had been assigned to my case. In my usual attempt to calm the pre-surgery jitters with wisecracks, I told them I really didn't have any tumors, but instead my ovaries had grown back. I asked them to help me fend off the tabloids when word of the scientific miracle broke, "The people from the *Enquirer* and the *Star* are sure to be here. They're really gonna want this story!"

We were all laughing and cutting up until the sedation began to take effect. Then I started to cry forlornly. I hadn't seen my doctor yet. I panicked, thinking he might miss the operation. When he did arrive, he wanted an explanation for the tears. I simply told him I was scared. His reassurances helped calm me down and I was wheeled off to the O.R. where he performed the surgery according to the scheduled game plan.

As always, I woke up with a nasal gastric (N.G.) tube running down the inside of my nose and into my stomach and a urinary catheter in place. The N.G. tube is used to pump the stomach fluid out and prevent sickness by keeping the system empty until the bowel is functioning normally again. I felt very uncomfortable and my stomach was really hurting. The surgery had produced yet another up-and-down abdominal scar from the incision. When the doctor stopped by to check on my recovery, the usual silliness surfaced once again. It was amazing how familiar such a complicated routine had become for me.

"How are you Nancy?" he asked.

Without saying anything, I grabbed the "smile-on-a-stick" a friend had sent me and put it over my mouth. It was a huge smile on a simple bit of cardboard glued to a tongue depressor—the perfect item for the cancer patient who tires of trotting out her own smile for the endless "How are we doing?" medical personnel.

It was also a familiar tale the doctor told me afterward. I'd be switching to a new chemo, "You'll need to have a porta-cath put in your chest to get the chemo this time."

I was adamant, "No! I won't have one of those. Dave's mother died with one in her chest. Forget it!" I was picturing the tiny catheter tubing and cap that provide a "permanent" port for administering chemo and other medicines directly into the vein— even though it would save me from the I.V. needles I'd inevitably need, the thought of a porta-cath sticking out of my chest gave me the creeps!

He ignored me, "You're going to need it. You'll be getting your chemo at home." Noting my disbelief, he continued, "We're giving you this drug, Taxol, at home. As long as it's working and effective, the treatments will continue non-stop. Maybe even for a year or two. You'll have a nurse come to the house once a month and administer the dose. You'll be back here in Baltimore in August for your first one, just to make sure you can tolerate it, but then you're on your own."

His mouthy little cancer patient was stunned into (temporary) silence. I'd never envisioned such a convenient setup.

⚬

Before the first treatment could occur I had to have the catheter port inserted, the device I came to refer to as my microphone (because of the long, rubber tubing attached to it). It came in handy for "mic checks" at boring staff meetings and at other times when I felt a diversion was necessary. It was a double Lumen Hickman catheter, designed for two incompatible drugs to be administered at the same time if needed. It would help preserve the veins in my arms, given the long haul I could be in for with the prolonged chemo.

The first Taxol treatment would take place at Sinai in August, but I needed to find a home health care nurse in Morgantown who could help me with the subsequent doses. The nurse would show me how to maintain the dressing on the catheter port and help me with the treatments I'd be getting every twenty-one days at home. I picked a company out of the phone listings and left a message with the answering service. When a woman named Connie returned the call, my curiosity was aroused. "Connie who?" I asked. It turned out "Connie" was a woman I already knew.

"I'm going to take care of you," she explained comfortingly.

She showed me how to "glove up" to change the dressing, making sure the port site stayed as germ-free as possible. My mission was to protect this little gizmo that served as a lifeline of sorts. It was strange to look in the mirror and see it dangling from its mooring in my chest—yet another metamorphosis on my journey of survival.

Connie asked me to think about what I'd like to do to pass the time during my treatments, "We're going to be together for the six-hour-long infusion every month. We could watch videos, quilt, whatever sounds good to you." When I told her I didn't know how to quilt, she announced it was high time I learned and told me to hunt down a quilt top.

The one person I knew who could help me out was Dave's grandmother. Sure enough, when I visited and explained my dilemma, she slipped into a bedroom and returned momentarily with the item in question. "I bought it from a lady out in the country near Fairview," she explained, "It's a double wedding ring pattern." This was the beginning of my "Taxol quilt."

On August 5th I returned to Baltimore for the initial Taxol treatment. I chose my seat in a roomful of recliners and I.V. poles and was hooked up without incident. The Taxol slowly entered my body over the course of six hours. The three pre-medications I was given, Decadron, Zantac, and Benadryl, protected my stomach and held off the nausea. Even so, I dipped into my ever-present supply of red-hot jawbreakers—the "atomic fireballs" that combatted the awful metal taste the chemo left in my mouth and the queasy feeling that crept up my throat. Somehow, and unbelievably, I'd drifted off to sleep during the infusion.

When I awoke Dave asked if I was feeling okay. I felt confused, "How come I'm not getting the chemo?"

"You are," he pointed out, "You've been getting chemo for the last half hour."

I was baffled. How could I be having a treatment and *not* be throwing up? No matter the reason, I became very emotional in my appreciation. Later, in the privacy of the ladies' room, I dropped to my knees and thanked God. To me, getting my life-saving medicine and not puking my guts out in the usual fashion was nothing short of a miracle!

I even began to feel hungry. Dave asked, "What sounds good?" After a second or two I mentioned a toasted cheese sandwich. Yeah. A sandwich and some peaches. That should hit the spot. For most people, especially Dave, almost anything from the Sinai Hospital cafeteria would hit the spot. I can even remember him bragging to a man about Sinai's great food while I was talking with the guy's wife about her cancer. When the food came I ate it with gusto, not with the approach I was familiar with: peck at this and that, then gag.

Remarkably, my long-held association between chemo and killer nausea and vomiting was fading. I was eating and even laughing during the process. There was a sweet little woman who was talking to Dave during her rehydration. Her name was "Mrs. M." and she was fighting lung cancer. I wasn't near enough to hear their conversation but the mere sound of their laughter gave me the giggles. When she finished her hydration fluids, she stood up and said loudly, "Thank you Sweet Jesus!"

⨍

It was sad to see that once again, after just one treatment, my hair was falling out. This time I thought I'd be ahead of the game and shave it all off before I was left with nothing but a few desperate strands to contend with. I asked my future daughter-in-law, Jill, to help me out, "Your choice. The clippers to cut the hair or the vacuum to sweep it up?"

She turned me down, "No. I can't do this. Dave will be really mad."

I took matters into my own hands, shaving the top of my head and clipping an artsy looking strip down the back of my scalp. Then I went downstairs to find ("surprise") my husband.

"Dave, where's the laundry basket?" I asked, trying to get his attention.

Without looking up he replied, "It's on the dryer."

"Where?"

He repeated, "It's over there on the dryer."

"Daaave?"

This time he turned to look at me, "Oh my God! Nancy, what have you done? Why did you do that?"

I explained that it was going to all fall out anyway and I was just getting a jump on things. He led me out to the deck. I leaned over the rail and he shaved off the remaining hair.

Shortly after that, ugly little pimples and scabs started breaking out all over my head. They were so painful I couldn't even wear the new wig I'd purchased. (It was a cute little bob that I thought would perk up my appearance.) When I saw my oncologist on a follow-up trip to Baltimore a few weeks later, with a flourish I pulled off my scarf, tilted my bare head toward him and demanded an explanation.

"Take a look at this! What do you suppose is causing *this*?" I asked, half expecting to get the skinny on some rare drug side effect.

"What did you do?" he wanted to know

"I shaved my head, that's all," I replied innocently.

The cross-examination continued, "And during this shaving did you happen to have a guard on the clippers?"

Uh oh.

"It's called folliculitis. You've irritated all the hair follicles and gotten them infected. You're not going to be able to wear the wig until this heals up," he explained.

"I can't go to work like this! I can't," I pleaded.

"Hey, I'm looking at a very attractive woman with a beautiful scarf on her head. There's nothing wrong with that," he said, consoling me.

Eventually I was able to laugh about it and my fun-loving co-workers did too. They poked fun at me and called me "the pirate" because of the way I wore my scarf.

❦

In September I borrowed a quilt frame from a woman in my church and got things set up for my first afternoon of "Chemo and Quilting with Connie"—it sounded like a show you'd see on some obscure cable TV channel. Connie brought lunch for the two of us. We ate. We quilted. My six-hour-long infusion of Taxol seemed to pass quickly. I remember Connie telling me her fellow nurses were amazed by this new "at home chemo" procedure, which was breaking new ground on the local chemo scene.

Just as at the hospital, I slept peacefully through much of the infusion. And the greatest thing of all—I wasn't sick! I also needed continual infusions of magnesium and potassium because I still had trouble retaining them and didn't want another "P.M.S." stint.

I had the idea to write things on the quilt and to let friends and family write on it too. In one of the squares I wrote, "Taxol, Fireballs and Toasted Cheese," in celebration of the first chemo treatment I'd ever tolerated without getting ill. There's even one that says, "Hair Today, Gone Tomorrow." To further commemorate that joyful day I wrote on yet another square, "Thank you Sweet Jesus! —Mrs. M."

To Everything There Is a Season...

It was shortly after the second Taxol treatment that I began having trouble. My tongue would swell and I had to take Benadryl to counteract the problem. By the third treatment, in October '94, the response was extreme. The swelling reached my throat and I couldn't swallow.

Ultimately, the allergic-type reactions began to be too much. I could read the handwriting on the wall. It said my new friend Taxol and I would be parting company. Back in Baltimore my doctor recommended a substitute drug called "Topotecan." Unfortunately, because it was still an investigational medicine and I wasn't quite on my deathbed, it would take a lot of paperwork and luck to get my prescription approved.

Okay, so I wasn't on my deathbed, but I wasn't feeling well either. Ever since the June surgery I'd battled problem diarrhea. The situation was peculiar. It would hit me hardest at night. The bowel movements were bloody and full of mucous. I couldn't control them. This made it especially hard to keep working.

Outside the office I came up with still other coping mechanisms. I learned where all the bathrooms were located at the mall and conducted my shopping with an emergency strategic plan in mind at all times. Not even this disgusting condition was going to keep me from going out and living a "normal" life. I just had to be careful about where I was and for how long.

I complained to the doctor about my extreme symptoms and underwent a variety of tests. Finally it was confirmed. He could palpate a small growth in the bowel—the likely culprit in my own private whodunit. His decision was to do a biopsy. This meant spending a couple days prepping for the procedure. The bowel would have to be completely empty. The laxatives and enemas kept me running to the bathroom nonstop.

My sister Judy was in town for the week visiting my mom, who was sick and in the hospital. My mother suffered terribly from rheumatoid arthritis. The anti-inflammatory medications she took interfered with her red cell count and she sometimes needed transfusions.

Judy stopped by my place to wish me well the night before the big trip east. "How are you going to make the trip to Baltimore tomorrow if you're still dashing to the restroom constantly?" she asked worriedly. I'd envisioned taking towels and clean clothes and just winging it, but she had a better idea. "We'll take our Winnebago," she offered. It was a good plan.

These hills never look more lovely than in October when the leaves glitter like bright jewels on the trees. The colors that year were spectacular and the miles of forest-covered mountains between here and Baltimore made the drive seem more like a tourist adventure than a medical excursion. I spent the entire trip on the commode, looking out at the autumn scenery as it flashed past the tinted window, my porthole-like view of the outside world. "Judy, are you *positive* those truckers can't see in? It sure seems like they're looking in when they pass," I asked nervously, accepting her solid reassurance with just a sliver of doubt.

While it's impossible to say I was looking forward to the upcoming biopsy, I was eager for some answers. My situation had become somewhat desperate! At the office I'd developed a strategy to travel safely from my desk to the restroom. I called it "chair hopping." If I could proceed from one chair to the next, making momentary rest stops on my way to the bathroom, I could complete the trip without incident. In the meantime, it took all my concentration and a lot of "puckering" to keep from having an accident. These bathroom sojourns took place several times during each of my workdays. I think my co-workers assumed I went from chair to chair to keep from fainting.

We finally arrived at Sinai Hospital of Baltimore, where a nurse greeted me with an apology, "I know you're exhausted but you'll have to endure two more enemas before your procedure. How do you want to do this?"

Too exhausted to do anything but comply, I told her to give me a bed sheet and I would lie on the bathroom floor. When that ordeal was through I was eventually led into the exam room where an intriguing assortment of instruments was arranged before me. What fascinated me most were some giant cotton swabs measuring about eighteen inches long. Just before the doctor stepped in I asked the nurse if I could borrow two.

"This *is* what these are for, right?" I asked as he entered the room. His face had an expression of shock as he looked at me, a giant "Q-tip" sticking out of each of my ears.

"Yes Nancy," he said, sighing a no-nonsense sigh. "That's exactly what they're for. Now, let's get started. Turn around and lie on the table, grab onto the bars on the side."

"What?" I asked, stooge-like, "I can't hear you, I have these big Q-tips in my ears."

He tilted the table and I let myself start to slide off, laughing on my way. His tone became more serious as he picked up my hands and placed them on the bars, "Now hold on this time!"

In just seconds he was finished. He'd located the growth and snipped a small sample to be biopsied. I couldn't help think of the drawn-out, uncomfortable ordeal I'd been through to facilitate this quick procedure. He promised to rush the sample through pathology and have the results the next day.

"How did it get there?" I wondered out loud.

"The cancer can travel throughout your body," he explained. "Now, I want you to call me at three tomorrow afternoon. The best-case scenario is that this is ovarian. If it's colorectal cancer we've got another battle on our hands. Ovarian we can treat along with the existing tumors. Three o'clock, okay?" I agreed.

I was feeling antsy at work the next day. I watched the clock slog its way to noon and then told my boss I had to leave, "I think I need to go clear my head. I'm going to Coopers Rock."

It's a state forest just outside of town. There's a large rock out-crop there, jutting like a massive stone pulpit high above the Cheat River. The enormous camouflage of foliage can capture your thoughts and hide them from God himself. In the distance to the right you can see the local airport and further still, the WVU Coliseum, looking like a tiny stack of coins from the vantage point of the overlook. To the left is the Chestnut Ridge, a thick blue spine of mountain and powerful reminder of the enduring nature of things Appalachian. It's a part of the "Allegheny" Range—the Delaware Indian word for eternity.

I phoned Mom and Dad's place to invite Judy, "You want to go on a picnic?" She was game. We put on our ball caps, grabbed some sub sandwiches, put the top down on my little mauve-colored VW Rabbit convertible and hit the road. If I'd had my old hairdo I'm sure the breeze would have felt great blowing through it. I even took our new video camera, just for fun. It was an idyllic autumn after-noon, save for the menace in my gut that would soon be identified.

Up on the rock we stretched out and ate, basking in the bittersweetness of the fall air and allowing our gaze to follow the miles of mountain that quickly seduce one to daydreaming. Then my minister showed up. "Reverend Agnew, what are you doing here?" I wondered aloud. He explained that he'd stopped at the hospital to visit Mom and she told him we were out here, counting down the minutes until my biopsy verdict was pronounced. The three of us sat and talked for a while and enjoyed the sunshine.

When he left I made a suggestion, "Judy, let's pop over to the park, okay?" Chestnut Ridge Park is a place where hours of our childhood had evaporated under the summer sky. I caught numerous sunburns plunging in and out of the pond, splashing and playing with the other kids, celebrating the end of school for a glorious three months until it began again. On this anxious day Judy and I poked around in the water with sticks here and there, killing time.

After about a half hour I realized the designated time was near and we needed to get to a phone for the three o'clock call. We asked the woman at the park office if we could use hers. She agreed.

"Judy, it's got to be ovarian. It's just got to be ovarian!" I repeated as I dialed.

The doctor, sensing something odd, said, "Where exactly *are* you?"

"Oh, I'm up in the mountains," I explained, touching on our afternoon itinerary. Then he said what I needed desperately to hear, "It's ovarian cancer, Nancy."

I yelled to Judy, "IT'S GOOD NEWS! It's ovarian cancer!" The park lady looked bewildered as she watched us jumping up and down, a little victory dance at the news it was ovarian.

He said, "You know, we're still going to have to figure out your treatment since you can't tolerate the Taxol. Let's keep working on the Topotecan."

Feeling jubilant, Judy and I got the idea to go to the nearby stables for a horseback ride. Once there, I spotted a huge trampoline. "Why not?" we muttered to each other, and I hopped up to give it a go. I briefly questioned the wisdom of this, having the Hickman port in my chest and fighting the ongoing diarrhea and so on, but... life is short, right? I held the port with one hand, using the other to balance as I jumped wildly up and down, giggling hysterically, and waving to Judy, who was videotaping the event.

"Oh, Judy!" I screamed between laughs, "J...udy! My......Oh...My......My......pa...pants!" I felt myself lose control but was too helplessly giddy to stop. The trampoline was fun, but we craved still more activity, and in a matter of minutes had mounted a couple horses for a trail ride into the woods.

✢

I have cancer. That's a fact. But there was nothing going in my veins to combat it. Another fact. It was hard not to panic. I pushed the medical staff to do everything possible to get me the Topotecan. "Come on Nancy, you're not the typical cancer patient," they told me. "This drug is given on a 'compassionate need' basis, and face it, you're still going to work fulltime!" Yet another fact.

I kept in touch. I kept pressing for results, insisting, "I need this drug! What else can I do?" I even contacted a West Virginia senator, who told me if it were made available I could receive it at the Cancer Center here rather than driving to Baltimore. But nothing I did produced the desired outcome. I was up a creek without my chemo and worried the cancer was growing.

At Thanksgiving I took time out for my usual holiday reflection on life's blessings. True, I was grateful to be alive, to celebrate with Dave and my sons. To sit at the table filled with the traditional goodies and give thanks for my life's bounty. "Hello God. It's me, Nancy. I'm still here. Thanks!" And yet impatience paced the floor of my conscience.

Mid-December came. With the holidays approaching there was lots to do. I like to bake. I like to decorate the house for the season. While other women might have been hoping for tennis bracelets or bread machines, the big wish on my Christmas list was the drug that would help me survive.

One day a call came from Marilyn, a nurse at the Baltimore oncologist's office, "We have a Christmas present for you Nancy."

"I'm approved for the Topotecan?" I asked excitedly.

"No. We don't have your approval yet, but we do have another drug for you. It's called 5 FU. Your doctor doesn't want you going any longer without chemo."

I was curious, "What about side effects?"

Marilyn replied, "It's actually tolerated pretty well. Once a month you'll receive a continuous four-day infusion."

"Really?" I asked skeptically.

"Yep. We want you to start tomorrow," she said, enthusiasm in her tone.

My older son Greg was just wrapping up the fall semester at WVU's Law School and was scheduled for knee surgery to repair some torn cartilage. "I can't start it tomorrow," I explained, "I need to be there for Greg's surgery."

She assured me I could get the chemo *and* be with him, "The chemo unit is only a little bigger than a tin of band-aids. It will have a thin line that hooks up to your port. You'll store it in a small pouch you can wear around your waist. It's so simple, you'll be walking around for four days and not even know you're getting chemo."

She was right. My friends at work bought me a neat little leather fanny pack to conceal my medical gadgetry. Except for the occasional dispensing noise, like the sound of film automatically advancing in a camera, I was inconspicuous and free to roam. I was at the hospital with Greg. I went shopping. I ate in restaurants. I went to a Mountaineer basketball game, telling everyone in sight, "Look, I'm getting chemo! I'm at the game and I'm getting chemo. It's the coolest thing." I'd pull back the collar of my shirt and show them the port site, "Isn't this neat?" We vacationed in Hilton Head. We did lots of things other people wouldn't think of doing under the circumstances, but it was so easy to live a normal life with the 5 FU.

The chemo was usually delivered to me at work. It came via rush shipment to the hospital receiving dock and then I was supposed to get a phone call notifying me of its arrival. Often impatient to know that it was safely on the premises, I'd walk down to the dock and question the guys, "Have you seen my little box of chemo? It says, 'Attention Nancy Lofstead' on it." They'd shuffle a few crates around nonchalantly picking through the cartons until they spotted my precious batch of 5 FU.

By January of '95 I was back in Baltimore for another exam. My oncologist was leaving to work at Dartmouth and wanted to introduce me to the new physician who would be taking over my care at Sinai. When the new kid showed up I viewed him as just that.

"How old are you?" I said, doubting this young man's credentials because of his wet-behind-the-ears appearance.

"I'm thirty-five," he replied confidently.

Hmmm...he doesn't look much older than Greg, I thought, rolling the thought around in my head to see how it would settle. "How are you going to handle me?" I challenged him, adding a little white lie. "My other doctor sings for me. Are you going to sing to me too?"

"First of all, I think I can handle you," he said, and then paused for a moment, "And I think I do a pretty good Elvis impersonation."

He wanted to check my port but I jokingly said I never showed my port on the first "date." Then I told him Elvis could wait until our next visit and we managed to get down to business.

The doctors agreed that the small nodule in the bowel could be removed. I resisted. After all, we'd only given the 5 FU a month to get to work. "Let's wait and see what the chemo does," I countered. They went along with my plan but only on the condition I'd come back in the spring for a follow-up exam. Deal. I'd be there.

Good little patient that I am, I kept my promise and reported to my new doctor in Baltimore in March for the evaluation. "You know, I really think we need to take that out," he concluded after looking at the results of my most recent M.R.I.

I immediately started the dickering process, "Okay, but can we do it here in the office? Outpatient?" He explained that wouldn't be possible. I'd have to be put to sleep. "Okay but I'm going home the same day. As always, I'll want the procedure on Friday so I can go back to work on Monday," I forewarned him.

"Well, we'll just have to wait and see if there's any bleeding. If it's excessive you'll need to spend the night here," he cautioned me, and proceeded to set up the appointment for the second weekend in April, which happened to be Easter.

On Good Friday I found myself back on the operating table. Dave, Mom, Dad and I had made the trip over the day before so I could prep overnight. We checked into a nearby hotel where I spent most of the time on the commode, having drunk the usual fifty-gallon barrel of bowel preparation to clean me out. The three of them flipped through TV channels searching for the kind of ideal diversion that always evades those caught in periods of anxious waiting trying to pass the time.

On that Friday morning I was led down the hall near the O.R. and asked to take a seat. "We'll take you to surgery in a little bit," someone assured me.

I was a tad nervous, "Don't I get a pre-op shot or anything?"

"No, we'll take you in there in just a moment," a nurse explained. My doctor approached and asked how I was feeling.

"Fine," I lied, as I was handed a couple little pills that were supposed to prevent stomach irritation.

"Good. If you're ready to go, let's head on in," he said.

He walked beside me as I shuffled down the hall in my little green slippers. I was holding onto my port and eagerly waiting for someone to feed a relaxant or sedative into it. Once in the O.R. I climbed up onto the table and watched the staff strap electrodes all over me. I clung to the port and waved the little tip, "I'm ready for my martini!" As usual, the more nervous I became, the more joking I did. I don't recall what I'd told them, only that they were laughing. My compassionate new doctor calmly held my hand as I slipped off to sleep. It became a trademark gesture he'd repeat in subsequent procedures.

An hour and a half later I awoke in recovery to the news that the tumor he'd removed was rather large but everything had gone well. In a short while I was seated in a chair, too groggy to keep my head upright, but clear-minded enough to insist on heading home. At half-past noon we were on our way.

I had some mild bleeding and discomfort on the way, but I was able to stretch out in the back seat and get some sleep. That evening the doctor called to check on me. "I'm having quite a bit of bleeding at this point...and some clots," I informed him. He said that was to be expected, given the size of the tumor, much larger than the M.R.I. had indicated. "Just how big was this thing?" I wanted to know. I was as surprised as he was to learn that the growth taken from my body that morning was nearly as big as a BASEBALL! He told me he couldn't believe that I had been as functional as I was, housing a tumor with a four-centimeter diameter in my rectum. Truthfully, neither could I!

He encouraged me, saying I should recover very well, and that he was glad the process was over with. He reminded me to stick with a liquid diet through the next day. I found it impossible to comply. I was so hungry I started snarfing down crackers. My neighbor Linda observed this defiance and said, "That doesn't look like a liquid diet to me—that stuff's really going to hurt coming out!" I was starving and couldn't help myself. Ultimately, I was just fine. On Sunday I devoured a delicious Easter dinner. Pleased with my resilience, I reported to the office on Monday without problems or difficulty.

I continued my monthly 5 FU treatment. I even had to sleep with the pack during the four-day infusion. It was a bit uncomfortable, but at that point it seemed a small sacrifice to make because it was so user-friendly! I'd taken up roller blading. I relished the fact that I could get my chemo as I skated long, rhythmic laps around the Coliseum. I loved breathing in the fresh spring air and being active. I'd play some really upbeat music on my Walkman to keep me fired up. Janet Jackson tunes, stuff like that.

At one point I had a bit of a scare with the 5 FU fanny pack. I'd reached in to check the chemo level and immediately noticed a dark fluid apparently oozing from the side of the cartridge. I thought the chemo or the battery must have been leaking into the pouch. As I pulled it out for closer inspection the distinct smell of chocolate caught my attention. There, squished and melted in the bottom of the pouch was a severely deflated Hershey's Kiss!

I was looking forward to the 1995 Relay for Life, but by late spring I had started having a strong adverse reaction to the 5 FU. I developed terrible mouth ulcers! I really wanted to be there, but that year it simply wasn't possible. Along with Connie, my chemo and quilting nurse, several people from work were planning to walk with me at the Relay, which, unfortunately, was scheduled during this period of my severe reaction to the chemo.

By the night of the Relay my mouth was so full of sores I could barely open it. My tongue was incredibly swollen. I telephoned the medical staff in Baltimore and mumbled enough words for them to figure out what was happening. My doctor ordered I.V. fluids to be administered at home, just to make sure I was keeping hydrated. He told me I'd have to stay home for at least the next three days.

When Connie came over late in the afternoon on the day of the Relay I told her I was sure I could make it if she'd agree to push the I.V. pole around the track for me. Even though I insisted that I be there, that I couldn't miss the Relay for Life—it had come to symbolize so much in my struggle—Connie stood her ground as my good nurse and kept me at home in bed (where I no doubt belonged!).

I was so excited about the Relay. It had really been well publicized and I was sure the turnout would far exceed the first year's. How disappointing to be lying in bed in my Relay t-shirt, watching the fluid drain slowly from the I.V. bag into my arm when, by rights, I should've been rounding the track in celebration of my ongoing existence!

My consolation was that Dave had captained a team and walked in support of me that year. Along with that, when the event ended, two of my "cancer cousins," Jane and Raymond, came by to give me a balloon and one of the commemorative Relay for Life towels that had been handed out to the cancer survivors. I dragged my I.V. pole and my swollen mouth out to the den where we all watched a videotape they'd shot that evening. I was secretly thinking, no matter what, next year I'll be there in person! (And I was!)

My dose was decreased to allow me to better tolerate the 5 FU and overall, the chemo was good to me. For nearly two years.

A Blue Coat

Finding a chemo that allows you to maintain your lifestyle *and* your hairstyle is a real plus. I can "fit in" if I still have my hair. I don't feel like an alien when I look in the mirror and see that I still have a few locks to style. To me, having hair means being able to go out in public without generating the obvious reaction, "Oh look at her. She must have cancer." It's not that I care intensely about what people think, but I do care about what *I* think. I feel better emotionally if I look okay. I'm a better fighter if I can stand in front of the mirror and see the physical representation of a relatively healthy woman. Hair is part of my cancer-fighting battle gear.

The American Cancer Society sponsors a program called, "Look Good, Feel Better." It's based on the theory that if you look okay, you'll feel okay. I'm reminded of the Billy Crystal character who says, "You look mahvellous dahling! And remember, it is better to look good than to feel good!" I try to look as nice as possible in the hope that feeling well will go hand-in-hand. I suppose in the back of my mind I'm rationalizing. If other people are saying to themselves, "Well, she looks pretty good," then maybe I've convinced them (along with myself) that I also *feel* pretty good.

Thinking it over, I've done some pretty funky things to achieve this "look" of health. At times my medications really affected my skin tone. I could end up with a really pasty complexion—not a speck of color in my cheeks. A friend told me at one point some gold eye shadow would brighten my face. I fell for it and started wearing this shimmery gold stuff to work. Nobody said anything one way or the other.

Then one day when I was feeling especially down. Sabra caught up with me just before a staff meeting.

"What's wrong Nancy?" she probed.

"Oh, I don't know," I bumbled. "I can't really pinpoint it. I guess it's that I look so awful. You know, I'm in front of the mirror and see that my skin looks just horrible."

"Well I'll tell you one thing. You've gotta lose that gold eye shadow," she willingly testified. "It's sure not helping matters."

"Really?" I said, knowing hers were the words of a true friend. The kind of friend who tells you when you've got toilet paper stuck to your shoe or something suspended from your nostril. "But someone told me it would help me look brighter and give me some color!"

As a cancer patient I often felt vulnerable to the power of suggestion. Had I followed many of those suggestions, I probably could have spent hundreds of dollars on clothes that people said made me look better, "This is a good color for you. It makes you look healthier. Remember, you need vivid colors to deal with that pale skin tone."

Occasionally following misplaced advice like that is the only explanation I have for some of the items that found their way into my wardrobe, especially in the early days after diagnosis. I bought a two-piece black outfit with huge fuchsia, yellow, and teal flowers on it. Yikes! The fact that I actually wore that gaudy get-up is a little scary in itself!

A friend once told me, "There's chemotherapy and there's retail therapy." She said shopping is what you do when you have to deal with the chemo. She was right.

I can recall trying at various times to perk up a bad day or lighten a bad mood with a little over-the-counter pick-me-up from ladies' wear. "I'm sure this new blouse will give me a boost," I told myself. My potassium might have been low, but it was a pretty new sweater, not more potassium, that got me back in the groove. If I thought red was the right color to fish me out of an emotional funk, then red is what I grabbed for my trip to the fitting room. It makes perfect sense to me.

I've recommended this shopping remedy to other folks over the years. I think it's beneficial—a regular retail tonic. Slipping into a new outfit and hearing someone pay a compliment like, "That's a great color on you! Where'd you get the new skirt?" can really lift your spirits. Retail therapy can soothe the sometimes-terrible effects of chemo.

There is one special purchase that stands out in memory. After the shock of my 1989 diagnosis in the spring and then a six-part series of killer chemo, I was glad to be around for a little shopping outing with my neighbor, Linda. Winter was coming and I needed a long dress coat for the cold months ahead.

What caught my eye was navy blue and just beautiful! It had leather and suede detail on the shoulders (remember, this is 1989). I fell in love with it, but tears came to my eyes at the realization that I'd never get my money's worth out of it, "Yes, I know it's beautiful Linda, but I won't even be around to wear it a second winter."

"Don't say that, Nancy!" she countered, "You're going to be here lots of winters."

The blue coat is still hanging in my closet.

My Fair Ladies

My mom's mother lived in Mannington, West Virginia, about a forty-minute drive from Morgantown. My siblings and I can recall the family visits to our grandmother throughout the year, but we especially delighted in our little overnight stays during the summer break. As luck would have it, her house was just a block from the town swimming pool and the fairgrounds, home to the spectacular Mannington fair. It gave us the sort of thrill some adults might feel on their annual Vegas getaway.

We loved to visit her each August at fair time! The smell of the fair wafted toward her front porch when the breeze was in the right direction. The odor was a combination of hot sugar spinning magically into cotton candy, corndogs bobbing in the fryer, popcorn exploding from the huge kettle poppers, perfectly groomed prize-winning livestock dining on fresh hay, and the gritty scent of motor oil from the midway rides.

A chorus of noise made it delightfully impossible to fall to sleep. There was the muffled drone of the man on the P.A. system constantly announcing something: Shmreith Fplgurg has won a prize and Blrhey Klartgegbeg should pick up her lost child at the entrance gate. There was the stream of traffic. Car motors purring sweetly along on the way in. Those same drivers honking, tired, trying mightily to be the first ones to leave when the grandstand show was *almost* over. And underneath it all, the hum of a thousand generators keeping the festive strings of yellow bulbs lit and the rides spinning and twirling—a collective squeal of elation wrung out of each turn.

The coins in my wallet raced to the money aprons of vendors selling snow cones, balloons, and all the cheap little trinkets children desperately need to own. Along with the other kids who buzzed around the fairgrounds, I, too, felt the sting of childhood's inequity—so much fun; so little time. Our inevitable group exodus at the end of the fair marked the start of the long desert of days between one summer and the next.

It was this collection of shared fond memories that prompted Carla and me to make a return visit to the fair in August of '95. I was taking my 5 FU and feeling well enough to head out for old time's sake. We drove to Mannington one sunny Friday afternoon, in a nostalgic mood and ready for some old-fashioned fun.

Along with all the "other" kids, we were eager to try out the rides. Did we feel more like whirling through the air on a little metal swing, outstretched under the spell of centrifugal force, or zipping headfirst toward the ozone, only to plummet back down an instant later? We chose the rocket planes, bought our tickets and got in line. That's when we noticed that the two boys in front of us had their hands stamped. Sensing we might be missing out on something, we pressed them for information. Turns out for about $11 you could get a stamp and ride all the rides you wanted for the whole day! After a long scrutinizing look, the lady in the booth refunded our ticket money and sold us the hand stamps. We were in business!

It had seemed like a good idea, rolling upside down in mid-air in a tiny steel rocket, and then progressing to a ride called the Scrambler. This one looked a little like a giant spinning tarantula or octopus, the huge "legs" flexing in and out from the center with a jerk of speed, the passengers seated in steel cages at outer extremes. The combination of the speed and the angle (and probably my poor physical condition) forced my body to press against Carla in a most uncomfortable squeeze.

"Move over! Nancy, move over!" she begged, trying to shout above the din of the midway.

My head, seemingly frozen at a forty-five degree angle from my shoulder, wedged against hers with an intensity that threatened to permanently reduce her hat size.

"Get off me!" she yelled in pain. "Move over! Get off me!"

But I couldn't budge. We'd become unwilling Siamese twins for the duration of the ride.

"I can't move, Carla!" I screamed in apology, at the same time trying to edge away from her. It was no use. The momentum of the spinning monster had us fused into the corner of the big metal holster like a couple of Twinkies smashed in the bottom of a lunch box.

We laughed and screamed, but by the time we were unstrapped from our shuttle seats, nearly stumbling back out into the midway, I knew I'd made a mistake. I'm not one to get sick on rides, but that day the Scrambler lived up to its name and nausea quickly overcame me.

Carla helped me make my way behind the Community Building, the place where housewives made an annual ritual out of oohing and ahhing over each other's delectable preserves and baked goods. All those pleasant memories were suddenly distant, given my impending problem.

I just sat there on the ground to rest, trying not to toss my cookies as the pungent smell of the nearby livestock barns filled my queasy nostrils. Drat! And we'd hardly hit the rides, I thought. The kid in me wanted to try them all, but the cancer patient needed to go get some rest and be out of all the noise and commotion. This posed a practical dilemma for me, as we'd just dropped more than twenty bucks on the ride stamps.

I wanted Carla to approach the same ticket woman and ask for a refund.

"I'm not going to do that!" Carla refused.

"Carla, just go over there and tell her your sister has cancer and you want a refund because I'm sick and we have to leave after only two rides," I urged.

"Forget it," she said, her tact firmly in place. "You want your money back, *you* tell her about the cancer."

It didn't happen. Neither one of us had the nerve to follow through. But the idea that I *deserved* to get that money back helped create a little monster in me that I'm not ashamed to introduce to you.

Back Off, I Have Cancer!

The Fair incident highlighted the fact that I could allow the cancer to "work for me." It's come in handy to get out of unpleasant tasks at work or to pad the results of my procrastination, "I'd love to help you all move that office furniture, but I have cancer." Or maybe, "I would have had that report done on time, but I have cancer."

Finding a place to park at Mountaineer Field can be quite a challenge, given the teeming masses of tailgaters and thousands of loyal spectators that cram the parking lots on football Saturdays. Even Dave's been known to resort to playing the cancer card when I'm not doing well, "Excuse me officer, my wife here has cancer and it would really tire her out to have to walk the seventeen miles to the stadium entrance. Mind if we park here next to the team bus until after the game?"

Frustrated restaurant hostesses don't quite know how to respond to me. When they say there'll be a fifteen-minute wait for a table, *unless* we want to sit in the smoking section, I look 'em in the eye and say, "No problem. I already have cancer. What's a little cigarette smoke?" Like rabbits out of hats, tables have been known to magically appear.

Parking spaces. Restaurant tables. I suppose it's akin to an elderly person getting the last seat on the bus, or traffic stopping to allow a pregnant lady to waddle her way across a busy street. It's all about exceptions to the rules. I just figure if we cancer patients have to endure this thing ravaging our health, we might as well get a few perks, right? Somebody gets on my case? A simple declaration sets them straight, "Hey, back off. I have cancer!"

Survival of the Feistiest

Over the years I've been asked to speak to various groups and talk about being a cancer survivor. People have asked how I define that term. For me, it's simple. If you're still alive after being diagnosed with cancer, you're a survivor. How long we survive is just a statistic. The fact that we can, and do, is the miracle.

I was once asked to address a team of social work majors at the University. As it turns out, the afternoon presentation couldn't have been scheduled for a worse time. That morning a group of Medicare

Surveyors showed up at the clinic, unannounced. My boss was busy with patients and *I* was left to face the surveyors' interrogation. Picture a kid on her first day on the job at Wendy's when the health inspector suddenly shows up. Okay, it wasn't quite that drastic, but the experience turned me into a bundle of nerves for the rest of the day. I found myself having to order my "johnny-on-the-spot" co-workers to fetch various reports and copies of our written standards to keep the team at bay.

I felt depleted of anything resembling charisma *or* charm by the time I entered the classroom. As luck would have it, the young sponges pumped me for information—for everything from the shock of a cancer diagnosis to the impact on my sex life. "Suffice it to say," I told the especially attentive youngsters, "With intense nausea and vomiting, and a huge, tender abdominal scar, one learns that there are many means of expressing love." I also spent time with the less personal stuff.

"We're *all* terminal, you know." And it's true—none of us will get out of this alive. "Just because I have cancer doesn't mean I'm dying and you're not. The inevitable awaits each of us. When I was first diagnosed with stage four metastatic cancer, there were those who automatically thought I had one foot in the grave. I'd read I might only last another year and a half."

When I was asked to comment on the question of mind over matter in fighting cancer, I was happy to. I gave them my stock answer, which is also my core philosophy: surviving cancer is 80% or more attitude, assuming there's proper medical care and some means of psychological support.

⤟

There have been studies that show a strong positive link between surviving cancer and having a support system in place. This has clearly helped explain the anomaly of my survival. My husband, family, co-workers, church and friends have all helped bolster my spirits with their love and encouragement over the years. As a result, and out of gratitude, part of my personal mission has been to reach others dealing with cancer.

Along with another employee at the clinic, I lead a support group that meets twice a month. It's for women with cancer, no matter what stage of illness they're in. It's called "New Horizons." It's just an informal get-together for us to talk about whatever concerns we have and to share coping mechanisms and other little tricks of the trade that we survivors need to know about.

I don't think God would have kept me around for this long if He didn't have a purpose in mind. My understanding of that purpose is to minister to other cancer patients as much as possible. When I was first diagnosed there was a glaring absence of support groups in the community. I think there was only one and it met during the day, so taking part was not an option for me because I continued to work fulltime. Knowing how much *I* would have appreciated having someone to talk to prompted me to visit as many cancer patients as I could.

At one point there was a man in the hospital who'd been a high school classmate of mine. He'd been diagnosed with bladder cancer and one of his relatives asked me to speak with him. We met at a time when his children were visiting him in his hospital room. They explained that he'd decided not to go through with any chemo because he'd heard such horror stories about it. I acknowledged that it was certainly a personal decision and that everyone had the right to choose for himself. Then I said good-bye, but mentioned I'd stop in again after my chemo treatment the next day.

I was nearly out of the room when he stopped me.

"What? Wait a minute. You're going to have chemo and then you'll feel well enough to stop up here to visit me?" He seemed totally baffled.

I assured him that was the case.

"Swear to God?" he asked.

"Yep! See you tomorrow," I said and excused myself.

The next day I arrived and was greeted with his hearty laughter. "You really just had chemo?" he wanted to know, a look of disbelief covering his face.

I informed him that I was certainly no expert, but that a lot of good medicines had been developed to help people deal with the awful chemo side effects. "Not all chemos make you sick, you know."

He hadn't been told this before and was eager to get more information. It's not uncommon for patients to get bits of information and not the whole story. They may even assume, out of the same sort of medical ignorance that I had in the beginning, that everyone will respond to a certain chemo in the exact same way. Had I known more about cancer, I certainly would have asked my doctors to remove *both* ovaries back in 1983 after getting the "borderline potential malignancy" readout. My thought is that there wouldn't have been an ovary to host the cancer six years later. But then there's no such thing as the tooth fairy, and in the cancer business there's no looking back.

I enjoyed visiting patients. I'll always remember meeting with a man who had brain cancer. He was a dentist. His daughter was a friend of mine and had asked me to please come and talk with him. Dave and I drove to their home and waited in the living room while the family finished dinner.

"Don't let me ramble, Dave," I reminded him, feeling a bit nervous about this particular visit because it was not the patient who'd invited me. "Stop me, give me a signal if I start to ramble, okay?"

"You'll be fine," he said.

Shortly after the conversation began (if you could call it that), I started to sweat it. This is going to be a wash, I thought to myself. It's obvious he doesn't want to talk about the cancer. When I asked the man how he was feeling, he said only, "Fine." Fine?? The guy was facing *brain cancer*, of all things!!

Meanwhile Dave was deep into a conversation about sports with my friend's husband, who was a college coach. I felt myself struggling to fill the dead air so I focused on having a dialogue with his wife. At some point I mentioned that I often lived on red Jell-O and tea right after chemo. It was as if I'd waved a sparkler in front of him.

"I DO TOO!" he interjected.

That small piece of information put us on a roll. The red Jell-O was the icebreaker we needed to make a connection. Suddenly he trusted that even though I am a woman with ovarian cancer, I might have some idea about where he was coming from.

I often fear I'll say the wrong thing to someone who's already feeling vulnerable and sick. I never offer advice. I don't represent myself as any sort of medical expert. I'm just a person who's doing her utmost to survive cancer and help others do the same.

❧

One day at work a social worker named Lisa called me from next door at the hospital. After a quick hello she launched into what must have been for her, a routine-sounding request, "We have a patient who has ovarian cancer and I'd like to introduce the two of you. I think that…" I stopped her when I thought she might have mistaken me for someone else, perhaps another social worker.

"I'm speaking with Nancy Lofstead, right?" she asked, sounding a bit confused.

"Yes, that's me," I said.

"Well don't you have the support group for cancer patients?"

"I *am* the support group," I answered.

"Don't you have a group that goes to visit people in the hospital?" she went on.

"No. But when the oncology nurses call me and tell me someone needs my help I walk over during my lunch hour and visit the patient," I explained.

She was taken aback and invited me to pop over and meet her in the third floor lobby so we could sit and talk for a bit in person. I accepted. After introducing herself, she apologized for the misunderstanding. The fact is she wasn't the only one to make that mistake. We had a good visit and stayed in contact afterward.

By the following year Lisa had formed "Facing Forward," a support group for persons living with cancer. She led the group, along with Kelley, a Cancer Center social worker who wanted to offer more help to her oncology patients. They asked me to join.

"Okay," I said, adding a condition to my agreement, "I'll join you. But the first boo-hoo and I'm outta there!" I had no intention of being part of a group that only got together to mourn in unison. *Of course* cancer is heartbreaking, gut wrenching, sad. I know that all too well. But what good would it do to get together if we weren't going to uplift each other and focus our energy on positive ways to beat this thing? I wanted to make sure the support group lived up to its name, "Facing Forward," and for the most part, it did. In fact, I became a faithful member.

By the time another year had passed Lisa and I were talking about one more way to serve cancer patients and their families. We thought it would be great if newly diagnosed folks could be paired up with cancer survivors to help them through that especially tough time. Out of this discussion came the "Cancer Care Survivor Team."

We got excited about the plan and produced a small brochure. We knew making those important survivor-patient connections could mean a huge difference. The idea was to offer emotional support and networking services during all phases of treatment. Everyone who became a member of the team underwent a training session at the hospital to learn how to educate patients and provide informational resources.

⁂

One thing I can't stress enough is to let go of the painful, negative experiences of life. Those things only burden us and eat up precious energy needed to fight the battle for survival. Let go. Let go. LET GO! It's probably one of the most important steps to take in freeing up the spirit. Without question, face forward!

Another important step? Whenever possible, be your own advocate and know what's happening. Ask questions and make sure you get explanations that make sense. Don't be afraid to ask a doctor or nurse to fulfill the "educating" part of their job description when it comes to strange-sounding medications and procedures.

Stay feisty and use humor! It's worked for me on more than one occasion. For example, one time when my hair finally grew back after chemo left me bald, I was chagrined that it returned in tiny, tight ringlets! It was so tight I couldn't run my fingers through it without getting them trapped in the little kinks. I figured I'd have fun with it because there really wasn't anything else I *could* do.

People would innocently ask, "Where'd you get your perm?"

"Oh, do you like it?" I'd ask, and then go on to explain it was called "Curls by Chemo." "You don't even have to go to the salon or smell that nasty perm solution. You just show up at the hospital and let them hook you up to an I.V. And the really great thing is, the health insurance pays for it!"

People would also inquire about my chemo regimen, "Nancy, how many more treatments do you have before you're finished?"

Knowing I'd probably always be on some sort of chemo, I'd joke with them, "Well apparently I made a mistake on my insurance forms and signed up for the lifetime plan!"

Hearing from survivors I've supported is one of the most rewarding feelings I know. One woman said she'd decided to go ahead with a prosthesis after I encouraged her to do what was best for her. It made her feel more confident about her appearance and less like a victim of a disease. Another wrote to say that my stories about roller blading around the WVU Coliseum with my chemo fanny pack inspired *her* to be out in public. She went to the Coliseum just to walk a few laps, but prior to that she'd felt embarrassed and ashamed about her cancer and a bald head that unmistakably advertised her condition.

One time I met with a brave young girl who was fighting for her life. She was only about twelve or thirteen, a tough age to navigate even without cancer. I remember sitting across from her at her home as we visited. The chemo had taken her hair but not her determination. As we talked I noticed she kept reaching up to scratch her scalp through the wig.

"Aren't those wigs uncomfortable?" I whined.

She agreed, seeming pleased with my expression of empathy.

"If you want to, just take the thing off," I suggested, "I've been bald too, *I* don't mind seeing your bare head."

Before I'd finished the sentence she'd grabbed the wig and tossed it aside like a magazine she'd tired of reading. It was a relief to me that we'd found some common ground despite our age difference and the conversation could really open up. Today that girl is a grown woman—a proud survivor who reminds me that anyone can be struck with cancer, and anyone, regardless of age, can put up a good fight.

When I spoke at a cancer survivors' luncheon one year I carefully choreographed how I would step back from the microphone after my little talk and slip through a door just behind the podium. Once there, I'd yank off my wig and pop on my baseball cap. Then I'd do away with my pretty blouse and show off the t-shirt I was wearing underneath. I'd seen it advertised in a catalogue aimed at cancer patients. On the front it said, "Hair by Chemo," and on back, "Not by Choice." The design featured a comb and scissors in a large circle with a line through it.

The time came for my big encore as I was wrapping up my talk. "Now this is how most people see Nancy Lofstead, the working professional," I explained coyly. "Give me just a minute and you'll see how I look at home."

The plan was to then burst back into the room through the door and watch their eyes pop out over my sudden transformation to Nancy Lofstead the cancer survivor. But even the best-laid plans can go awry. And they did. The door had locked behind me. I charged down the hall a bit and tried that door. Locked! I was forced to speed all the way around the corridor, finally entering from the main doors at the rear of the huge banquet room. Panting and perspiring, and facing their backs, I yelled to the audience, "Here I am! It's me! This is how I usually look." (Okay, without the sweat beads and thwarted look.)

All in all maybe the flaw in my scheme served to illustrate my core philosophy. If you're not the fittest, at least be the feistiest! Somehow I think Darwin would approve.

CHAPTER 4

Dance Lessons

1996 - 1997

The Health Benefits of Carrots

There'd been heavy rain and some flooding in the state in 1996. The Monongahela River, carrying barges packed full of gleaming black West Virginia coal, snakes its way through town on the way to Pittsburgh, some seventy miles north of here. There it joins its two river cousins, the Allegheny and Ohio.

During the green months, rain-swollen creeks skipped down the hollows and fed the river gulp by gulp until it seemed the "Mon's" murky belly was bulging. That fall the leaves were effervescent and brassy, due to "the right mix of water and sun," the experts proclaimed, a combination mountain people know as intuitively as when to harvest the ramps (those wild, smelly green onions).

I felt flooded too, with mysterious, unstoppable tremors that would overtake my entire body on occasion. They were followed by vomiting episodes and then a subtle return to normalcy. No one could determine what caused these strange occurrences. They usually happened at night, right after dinner. There was some speculation that the port had become infected, but I didn't have a fever and the blood tests and port cultures came back negative. The other diagnostic tests left us empty-handed as well.

The Easter week brought with it a strange case of déjà vu. I'd been having more instances of serious diarrhea throughout the early spring. My doctor's exam proved another bowel tumor was wreaking havoc with my system. He could palpate it, and thought it was smaller than the one he'd removed on Good Friday the previous year, but he wanted to get it out before it became unmanageable. Dave and I made the trip to Baltimore on our own.

Odd as it may seem, I underwent yet another bowel surgery on yet another Good Friday. The oncologist removed a mushroom-shaped growth attached by a stalk-type growth. He cut the tumor as close to the base as he dared, not wanting to risk a perforation of the rectal wall, and hoped more chemo would reduce whatever was left.

On the way home we stopped in Cumberland, Maryland for a bite to eat at the Bob Evans restaurant. We often did this sort of thing driving back from medical check-ups in Baltimore—dropping by a smorgasbord or Chinese restaurant, or maybe hunting for shoes at the outlet mall, or browsing through one of the antique shops that can be found along the interstate. Sometimes these stops were just the right diversion from a bad news diagnosis.

I remember various phone calls to Carla on days like these. "Well, it's not good. He says I'll need surgery/the cancer's spreading/the tumor marker's up..." whatever the case may have been.

"But where are you *now*?" she'd ask, sensing from the sound of cash registers or dishes clanking that we were not in a medical office, sagging under the weight of a diagnosis.

But this day was different. I recall shuffling across the parking lot and into the restaurant, hunched over in agony. We called ahead to Morgantown to make sure there'd be a prescription of pain medication ready to pick up at the pharmacy when we got back. That medicine helped me function the rest of the weekend. I used those couple of days to rest up, enjoy Easter Sunday, get back on solid foods and return to work Monday.

Soon matters had become much more serious than merely handling the oral discomfort the 5 FU had dealt me the year before. While the mouth ulcers subsided with the reduced dose, a serious bi-product was that the CA-125 tumor marker was now rising again. My doctor suspected the cancer cells were becoming resistant. A CAT scan showed the appearance of some enlargement of a few small tumors in my pelvis and abdomen. The shaking instances were happening more often. These jitters were so violent that I shook as though I were freezing.

⁂

Among other things, I was determined to be at my son's October wedding in Philadelphia. The date dangled in the distance like the proverbial carrot that I would not allow to leave my periphery. I'd been there when the boys graduated from high school. I had just watched Greg finish law school and Geoff graduate with his master's degree. Those carrots had come and gone. Part of the trick in this survival game was to keep lining up new carrots.

Sometimes they were simple carrots, like a family outing to Coopers Rock over the Labor Day weekend—just a laid-back time for us to enjoy hanging out as a family. Other carrots were major family events. One such carrot was "Greg and Jill's wedding." I would need this carrot even more than expected when I learned the cancer had spread to my bones.

That year I was thrilled to take part in the annual Relay for Life cancer fundraiser, but I recall not being able to take a deep breath as I made my way around the track. There was a slight pain in my ribs, but I told myself, somewhat unconvincingly, that I must have just pulled a muscle. It was a pain like the ones I'd felt climbing into the stands to watch Mountaineer basketball.

Of course, as a cancer patient I was aware that *my* aches and pains might be nothing other than what the average healthy person feels. Besides, I wasn't in enough pain to warrant the conclusion there was something terribly wrong. By the same token, anytime some little nuisance nudged at me from within, I contemplated the frightening fact that there could be more cancer.

Days after the Relay I asked one of the therapists at work to give me the once-over and confirm it was indeed a simple muscle problem. Instead, his suspicions were roused and he urged me to have my doctor check out the rib pain.

By early summer I'd undergone a CAT scan *and* a bone scan. The bone scan is a relatively simple test. Two to three hours prior to the scan I was injected with a small amount of radioactive liquid. My understanding is that the liquid is then absorbed into the bone in the areas where there is active metabolism and the cancer has affected the bone density. I lay strapped to a narrow table, my whole body passing slowly and methodically through a tunnel-like scanner similar to the machine that produces a CAT scan. It takes about a half hour.

My tests that summer confirmed the cancer had, in fact, spread to the bone. The mystery of the pain in my right rib had been solved. Fortunately, there was just one spot. In fact, I could locate the small protrusion with my fingers. It was a tender little nodule but it produced lots of pain. The doctor put me on codeine to control the discomfort and allow me to rest.

I slept with a body pillow as well as some that were propped at strategic points around my body. Dave was in charge of pillow distribution and was careful to get me positioned for optimal comfort. The pain could be tremendous and at certain times throughout the summer I experienced it with nearly every breath.

�֍

Dave had a conference scheduled in Boston for late August so we made plans to fly in early and then drive down to Newport, Rhode Island, to spend a few days with his sister Bette and her husband Dave, a Navy Captain. We looked forward to having some fun and spending time on the beach.

Dave and I landed at Logan Airport. He ducked into the restroom while I waited for our baggage. A gentleman in a chauffeur's uniform holding a placard that said "Lofstead" caught my attention. I thought to myself, what could he want with us?

As I grew impatient waiting for Dave, the guy approached me and asked, "Are you Nancy Lofstead?"

"Yes," I replied, adding skeptically, "And who are you?"

"I was sent by Captain Dave Ryan, your brother-in-law. Is your husband here?" I was stunned. How'd he know me? "My car's out front. Where is your luggage?" he asked.

That ended up being the $64,000 question. Only Dave's golf clubs had plunked down the conveyor. Our luggage was nowhere to be found and we had to wait for it to be delivered later on.

The man took the clubs and put them in the trunk of a limo!!! We were flabbergasted. "Right this way," he said, ushering us into the back where Bette and her husband Dave were waiting to surprise us. What in the world was happening? Here we were, just minutes off the plane, sipping champagne and eating strawberries and elegant little chicken salad croissants. Bette's husband happened to be hosting a Caribbean cultural music festival with his brother. The rented limo was part of the promotion, so they decided to make the most of it and incorporate it into our visit. On the hour-long drive to their house we traveled along the coast and looked at the beautiful mansions that line the route. This was turning out to be an even more delightful get-away than we'd expected.

Dave and I had never been in a limo and now it appeared to be at our disposal for the duration of the trip! We took it to dinner at a great little restaurant on one of the islands. The experience was right off "Lifestyles of the Rich and Famous." The limo driver sat attentively outside while we ate. On the way home Bette and I climbed up to the moon roof like a couple of twelfth-graders on prom night. We stood waving and singing golden oldies, having a blast.

Dave rented a car to drive back up to Boston for his conference after the four of us had spent a few days together in Newport. I stayed behind to enjoy some R and R with my sister-in-law. Bette and I whiled away our afternoons relaxing at the beach. I was enjoying the company, the scenery, and the wonderful change of pace from work and chemo.

On the day Dave arrived back from Boston I had a tremor. It started with a bad headache and chills, but quickly escalated. Bette was puzzled, "It's so hot. How can she have the chills?" Dave put me in bed and dealt with the situation as best he could. Bette repeated a foreboding phrase, "This isn't good. This isn't good at all!"

She was right. Although the shaking episodes did not include enough combined symptoms to make us think there was something deathly wrong, we were truly baffled. After what had been, for the most part, a terrific vacation, we prepared ourselves to learn the worst when we left for home, knowing the results of the CA-125 (tumor marker) would be waiting to greet us.

Once back in Morgantown, word came from Baltimore that my tumor marker had not merely gone up. In fact, it had doubled, from 150 to 300. With an urgent tone the nurse who bore the bad news said, "Nancy, we have to get you on another chemo NOW!"

When I asked about the drug I'd be getting, she told me it was time for the Topotecan, which was now available "on the shelf" as they say in the pharmaceutical world. It was no longer restricted to use by patients on the basis of compassionate need.

"Okay," I replied.

"We need to start you on it right away," she added.

To her dismay, I politely refused, "No thank you."

"Don't you understand what I'm saying?" she asked.

"Well, I'll tell you this much, and you can pass it on to my doctor. If I'm dying, I'll take the chemo. If I'm not dying, I'll be attending my son's wedding wearing my *own* hair. I don't want to be sick on that day!" I explained, adding, "I will not have this chemo just now. You can go tell him I said so."

"Just a moment," she said, putting the call on hold to go speak with the doctor.

She came back to the phone shortly, "He says you can start the treatments after the wedding."

"Thank you," I responded, "I have a life! I'm in charge. It's my cancer!" I may be living from one carrot to the next, the way some people live from paycheck to paycheck, but in spite of my cancer, I DO have a life!

On one frightening occasion I was in the bathtub when a tremor took over my body. Dave wasn't home at the time. I phoned my next-door neighbor Linda. No answer. I called my sister-in-law, Becky, who lives nearby. Again, there was no answer. Finally, when I dialed my friend Jan, a voice greeted me through the line. I could barely speak and make myself understood, "JJJjaaannnnn. Ppppllleeease ccccommmme hhhhellllppp mmmeeeeee."

It would be impossible for me to make it out of the tub to unlock the door for her so I struggled (and finally succeeded) to stammer out the security code that would let her into the house through the garage. As the call disconnected, I sensed her panic, and indeed, felt my own deep sense of desperation.

Jan raced over to the house, ran into the bathroom and found me shivering uncontrollably, even though the water was nearly scalding. The situation agitated Winston, our Boxer. He paced nervously just outside the bathroom. He cried when it seemed that Jan might be hurting me as she pulled me out of the tub. Somehow Jan managed to put me in bed, where, as a last resort, she laid on top of me, literally covering me with her own warmth and body weight to subdue my shuddering.

It would not be the last time these dreaded tremors robbed me of control over my body. I fought them. I fought the cancer that crept around inside me, leaving its mark here and there. I fought it with drugs. I fought it with my will. From the beginning I'd made up my mind: I *would not* go gently into that good night!

⁂

I made it through most of September and was counting the last few days before my exciting debut as mother of the groom, but I still battled the instances of shaking and then throwing up. It was determined I needed a CAT scan at the end of the month, before the wedding. It would help the doctors with their decisions about my chemo.

I really hated CAT scans. In actuality, I hated the prep. On this occasion I was to have *both* a mammogram and scan in the same day. The CAT scan was to be at the Mary Babb Randolph Cancer Center here in Morgantown and the mammogram at the adjacent Betty Puskar Breast Care Center. Carla accompanied me and saw first-hand how I handle my little nemesis (the CAT scan prep). I was supposed to be drinking a fluid preparation two hours prior to the scan, but I chose to take a drink then pour a drink down the sink…take a sip, pour out a sip. I looked around to see if I could spot any hidden cameras that might convict me of this devious maneuver.

When I walked back out to the lobby to greet Carla after the mammogram she complimented me. "You're really doing well! Look how much you drank," she said proudly, pointing to the reduced level in the container.

I whispered, "I poured it down the sink. I poured some in a garbage can back in the changing room too. No one will find it back there."

She was appalled, "Nancy, don't you realize you have to drink that stuff?"

"C'mon, who's going to know I didn't drink the entire two bottles? Besides, it gives me diarrhea," I answered, justifying my deceit.

∝

On the morning before the wedding Dave and I were cruising down the interstate on the way to Philadelphia when I became increasingly anxious. The fear of getting sick at the wedding or rehearsal dinner grew more intense with every mile. The last thing I wanted was to create a spectacle of myself with an episode of uncontrollable vomiting. The thought of embarrassing Greg and the family prompted me to pick up my cell phone and dial my doctor in Baltimore. I begged him for something to relieve the problem, "Please! I've just got to get through the wedding without this happening. Give me everything you have in your arsenal!"

He reassured me he could help and called in some prescriptions to my Morgantown pharmacy. One was Benadryl. Another was Phenergan, a powerful anti-nausea suppository. The third was Zofran, another anti-nausea weapon. Next I called Carla, who was leaving later in the day, and asked her to pick up the medicine and bring it with her to Philadelphia.

As the evening progressed, I happily checked off "rehearsal dinner" from the mental itinerary I'd drafted. By the grace of God, Friday night was nearly over and I'd managed just fine. Feeling confident as we came back to the hotel, I was pleased to see my sister and other familiar folks arriving. At nearly the same instant I turned to Dave and stuttered, "It's sssstttarting aaaaggainnn."

This was his cue that I needed the small electric blanket (throw) we always kept with us. Back in the room, he hurriedly plugged it in and draped it over me. Carla was with us and looked at me in disbelief, "WHAT is going on? Is this what she's been talking about?"

Dave said, "I want you to see what she goes through." Out of habit he grabbed the wastebasket for me and, according to the sordid routine, I emptied the contents of my stomach into it.

Carla was clearly distressed, "Oh, my God! How long has this been...?"

I interrupted, "Off and on for several months now. What am I going to do? The doctors don't know what's behind it—they can't find anything."

While the wedding party and other guests were probably resting comfortably, dreaming puffy white dreams of the wedding, I was up most of the night shoving suppositories up my butt, taking pills and carefully planning my strategy for getting through the big day. I prayed over and over in earnest, "Please God, let me get through this wedding without an incident." It worked. I don't think anyone there knew what I was going through.

It certainly doesn't show in the wedding pictures, where I look as proud and happy as any mom could possibly be, wearing an elegant coral-colored outfit. I wasn't feeling great when the time had come to shop for the wedding, but with the help of my sister-in-law Becky I managed to luck out and find it on the first try. It was the color that first caught my eye. I thought the coral-salmon tone could do wonders, given my current state. I needed something colorful and in just the right shade to help give me a healthy, vibrant look. It was a two-piece silk suit. It had a fringed scarf that wrapped around the neck and hung low in the back and met my knee in front. I'd hoped it would work well with the October setting and I think it did.

Greg and Jill chose a beautiful outdoor setting for the wedding. It was on the grounds of a gorgeous old historic estate. The rehearsal went fine, but when the forecast said it would be very cold the next morning they got worried about me and their grandparents and some of the elderly guests, and moved the ceremony indoors. Our minister friend from Morgantown drove to Philadelphia to perform the service. The walkway that led to the reception was bordered with the most wonderful mums. The lovely lawn and garden added to the beauty of the day.

As a precaution I'd clued in a few key people, "If you see me take off suddenly, it's probably because I have to go throw up." So at one point, when I needed to leave the reception all of a sudden, an entire troupe of six or seven people automatically followed in my wake. All of the stalls in the ladies' room were occupied, so I leaned over the sink, gagging again and again—someone's caring hands holding the fringed silk scarf out of the way. Fortunately, because I was a little gun shy about what might happen, I'd barely eaten anything, and didn't vomit after all.

At the reception, a pleasant surprise awaited me. When Jill finished the father and bride dance, Greg escorted me to the dance floor. Looking into the face of my handsome son, the spankin' new husband, our eyes were filled with tears as we danced to "Wind Beneath My Wings," the song he'd requested in advance for the mother and groom dance. In fact, someone told me later they didn't think there was a dry eye in the place, at least among those who knew what a long shot it was for me to be around for his wedding and even able to dance!

Afterward, the music picked up and I stayed out there, dancing the "Electric Slide" and making a failed attempt to dance the then-popular "Macarena" with my sisters.

And so it was that Saturday, October 5th came and went. I had gained the title of mother-in-law. Another "carrot" has assumed its place in history, I mused on the drive home the next day. My focus now shifted to the immediate future. Monday the 7th was the day I was to be introduced to Topotecan.

The Best-Laid Plans

According to schedule I showed up for the first dose of my Topotecan at the Cancer Center. Before the chemo began I received some anti-nausea medication. I then sat through the thirty-minute treatment and was sent home to rest. I was back at work the next day and then off to the Center again that afternoon to repeat the process. I was to receive the Topotecan as an outpatient on each of five consecutive days, running Monday through Friday. During the first week of the protocol I bargained with my doctor to reduce the infusion to four days to allow me to tolerate it better.

Twenty-one days later I got my next helping of Topotecan. I managed relatively well during the treatment week, but then it slammed me! I threw up a few times. I couldn't eat anything. In response, I developed what I now call the "yellow food diet." Over time it included such things as peaches, macaroni and cheese, pears, rice, potatoes. I was afraid of what anything of any other color might do to my system. Kraft macaroni and cheese became a comfort food for me, prompting many people to ask, "How can you eat that stuff?" I'm not sure. I only know it helped me get some nourishment.

In addition, the Topotecan made me incredibly constipated. I started out taking three Colace (stool softener) capsules a day to get some relief but there was no victory to be had. My doctor suggested I up the dosage to six capsules a day. "Deal with the constipation!" he instructed me. I took his advice. But when he later asked about my success, I told him I was still constipated but that the "commode aerobics" were going rather well. "What?" he asked, baffled and a little hesitant.

"Well, I figured since I'm spending all this time on the commode, I might as well be getting some exercise—you know, get the old heart rate up and see if I can produce the desired outcome." Prompted by his perplexed look, I went on to describe how I'd rock back and forth while seated on the toilet, moving my arms up and down and sideways in a rhythmic callisthenic. Not even this original bit of restroom choreography would produce anything more than a little musket ball. At the office Carla might casually observe me passing by her desk on the way into the restroom. A month later I'd emerge looking like a discouraged prospector.

"Anything?" she'd ask, glancing up from her work.

"Nope," I'd respond. "But when it does come it's gonna crack the porcelain!"

My hair was now abandoning me for the third time! It had thinned to the point that I wasn't comfortable going out in public without something covering my head, so I was forced to dig out my chemo hat collection.

Soon the nausea response increased dramatically. Topotecan turned out to be a nasty drug for me. This "mail order special" of chemos did not match the expectations I allowed to build during my long wait for its arrival. It was discouraging to finally receive the drug, only to have it knock me on my butt. I struggled to go to work. It was all I could do to head straight home after the infusions and slip into bed.

After just two treatments I was having trouble getting in to work each day. I just physically could not do it! I'd call the office and say, "I think I'm going to be late. I just threw up and am trying to get myself back together." It was an effort just to get my pantyhose on! Struggling to lift my leg and insert a foot into the hose, I could easily eat up ten minutes in the process.

I phoned the oncologist in Baltimore and explained my weakness and the daily struggle. I told him the drug was cramping my lifestyle. "You'll have to make the call on this one Nancy," I was told, "Don't expend your energy where you don't need to. Are you going to park in front of the house and walk up two steps? Or park in the garage and walk the thirteen steps up from the downstairs?" They were good questions. I did not want to supply the answers. I refused to admit that maybe I, not the chemo, might have to change.

I faced the same sort of physical struggle at work. I'd make the trip from the car to my desk in brief, excruciating increments. It went like this: Move from the car over to the curb in the parking lot, then to the bench in the lobby. Breathe. Rest. Elevator. Rest. Waiting Room. Breathe. Breathe. Breathe. Desk. Triumph. If anyone intercepted me with the "You okay?" question, I could only nod, too short of breath to speak even the single syllable response, "Yup."

Co-workers asked, "Should you be working?"

All I could say in response was, "I have to. It's a mental thing. I am NOT going to let this beat me!" I would not surrender to cancer or to its pesky cohort, chemotherapy. And so I struggled through the last days of October. Then came November, with its Thanksgiving holiday, awaiting as usual my annual counting of blessings. This year I could add my new daughter-in-law Jill to the list, and the gift of seeing my son walk down the aisle. But I could not offer thanks for a wonder drug that might have restored my relative good health.

Tap Dancing

Unfortunately, there is often bitter with the sweet. November proved this well. Periodic X-rays throughout the fall had shown the pleural cavity around my lungs was filling with fluid. Apparently the cancer has many ways of letting one know it's there. One of them is a pleural effusion. My doctor tried in vain to persuade me to have a thoracic surgeon do a tap to drain off the menacing fluid, but I was leery. The thought of such a procedure really scared me.

I'd consulted several other patients for their input. They all offered a similar warning. "Don't do it unless you have to," they cautioned, "there's always the risk of infection because the chemo's brought your white count down, and along with that, the whole lung can collapse." It was true the Topotecan was interfering with my white cell count—wreaking havoc with the little battalions of infection-fighters that were supposed to protect me.

In a state of denial (or just stubbornness?), I reasoned that because I wasn't having *too* much trouble breathing, and I was not symptomatic, the tap was more of a risk than I was prepared to take. "Let's just keep going with the Topotecan chemo a little longer and see what happens," I directed. I stood my ground and continued to take my Nupogen. Supplied through my home infusion company, Nupogen was supposed to bolster my white count. Knowing the importance of the drug made it just a bit easier to jab those syringes into my thigh each day for several days following chemo.

My doctor wanted to continue to monitor the fluid level in the pleural cavity by taking periodic chest X-rays. The tests revealed that fluid surrounding my lungs had reduced their capacity to function. An oncologist at the Cancer Center recommended weekly follow-ups on the problem.

In late November I agreed to another chest X-ray. That day was also a treatment day. I hand-carried the film from radiology to my doctor's office on the way to my chemo session. The plan was for him to read the X-ray and then catch up with me to discuss his conclusions.

So I was there getting my infusion when he joined me to announce the news I did not want to hear, "Nancy, we need to do a tap." I thought for a second, got up and did a tap. Literally. I tapped away on that tile floor, the heels of my brown loafers clicking away and the I.V. tubing swinging in response.

Seeing no reaction, I stopped and gave a polite curtsey. "You said to do a tap. Sorry, this is the best I can do," I explained, "I've never had any lessons."

English is not his first language. He didn't get my corny little joke. The nurses did. They turned and left quickly to hide their laughter.

I sat back down in the chair. He looked straight at me and repeated, "We need to do a tap on you."

Stubbornly, I resisted the suggestion, "No, I'm not going through with it."

"You know your lung can collapse. There's a lot of fluid in there!" he warned.

"I'm not having you stick a tube in my chest," I protested, "I can't go through with it."

He finally acquiesced. "All right Nancy. Have it your way," he said, turning and walking away.

That same month I did, however, consent to a blood transfusion. My hemoglobin was low and the scare over contamination in the blood supply had died down significantly since 1990. A transfusion seemed the best option to help me gain a little ground on the obstacle course I was traveling toward feeling well. I'd been getting the Topotecan four days a week every twenty-one days since early October. It was tough on me. I didn't eat well. I had little energy. The chemo did its best to deplete my red cell count.

Carla's daughter, Nicole, accompanied me for the transfusion. I took the chemo quilt with the good intention of adding some stitches during the two-hour-long process, but instead the quilt drew the interest of the many chemo nurses I now considered my pals. We chatted away and laughed. The quilt traveled back home looking just as it had when it left.

The bag of thick blood hung overhead and drained, drop by warm drop, through my port and into my eager veins. I thought it looked like salsa. Nicole said tomato sauce. Whatever its resemblance to menu items, one thing was certain. It made me feel great. My cheeks even showed a bit of color for a change. It was one much-needed kick in the butt.

In January of '97 I needed another kick. This time the doctor wanted me to have two units. I refused. Let's stop at one and see what happens, I proposed. He agreed. I reported as scheduled for the two-hour-long salsa feed. "Hey, is it just me, or does this blood look thick enough to be salsa?" I asked the nurses. And before they could finish rolling their eyes, I added, "Because I swear that last transfusion really gave me gas!" They rejected both assertions with a laugh, especially when Dave said he'd had a bit of gas too, without a transfusion or salsa.

Afterward I went home and felt somewhat better, but not with the same "shot in the arm" feeling that I'd experienced with the first one. I was forced to admit that the second unit was necessary and showed up for the sauce the next day. Since then I've had daily injections of Procrit given through my port. It's a handy-dandy red cell booster.

My doctor was remarkably patient with me. February came. I don't recall whether the groundhog saw his shadow or not in '97, but I can clearly recollect my doctor's ongoing look of concern. He wanted to tap the fluid in my pleural cavity. I'd been on the Topotecan since October. He'd been after me to have a CAT scan to see if the drug had affected the tumor growth. I flatly rejected each suggestion. Not only did I not care for the scan itself, the prep just did me in. I became so anxious over the thought of finding more cancer that I saw the test as a frightening game of medical roulette. I'd chosen not to play. He honored my wishes, or gave in to my insistence, I'm not sure which, and continued to monitor my tumor marker.

One day, after a lot of thought about the state of my health, I strolled into my doctor's office and found him seated at his desk, which faced away from the door. I walked up behind him and put my hand on his shoulder. "You've been a very good doctor, but I haven't been a very good patient," I said apologetically. "I've been doing some thinking. Let's go ahead with the CAT scan, and if you want me to do another chest X-ray, I will," I said, the humble tone of surrender in my voice.

Flabbergasted, as if I'd just announced he'd won a seat on the next space shuttle, he let his pen drop from his hand to the desktop with a definitive plop. "I'm ready whenever you are," he announced without looking up. He got the orders to the nurses and I finally underwent the scan the following week.

The test results gave us bad news. It showed tumor progression. There were several different masses in different areas. Compared to the scan I'd had just months earlier, in September, there was definite progression. "We have to get you off this," he concluded, referring to the Topotecan. Apparently the drug wasn't doing anything for me.

I couldn't help thinking, what a waste! In the end, I hadn't lost *all* my hair with the Topotecan, but it had thinned so much I had to stick with my hats. No wig this time. Hats. That entire struggle with the vomiting, constipation and fatigue, it knocked my socks off, and there were still masses! I kicked myself for being so stubborn. If I'd taken the CAT scan earlier as the doctor had suggested, we would have known about the tumor progression and I could have switched off the Topotecan and onto a new drug that may have slowed the trend. Even so, the experience hasn't changed the way I operate when it comes to dictating (in part) what my own care will include.

I was told my new drug, Navelbine, would be tolerated fairly well. I was relieved and took my first dose in March. The Navelbine was easily administered at the Cancer Center during a relatively quick infusion. I just showed up one day a week for three weeks in a row, and then took a week off before resuming the process. Not bad! I jokingly referred to it as the "navel bean"—this chemo that spared my hair from the terrible fate inflicted by the previous therapies.

As time went on, I didn't fare as well as my hair did on the Navelbine protocol. After the second treatment I had a vomiting spell. It sensitized me to the point that I didn't want to go in for another session.

I forced myself to show up for the treatment, but once there, when the nurse approached and said, "You ready?" I had to admit that I was not.

I pulled my legs up to my chest and wrapped my arms around my knees. "I can't do it Rainey!" I said, my eyes filling with tears.

"Okay then, we won't do it," she said calmly. "Can I get you anything? Want a relaxer?"

"Whattya got?" I peeped.

"Ativan. Valium. Does one of those sound good?"

I nodded. She got me a drink of water and a small milligram dosage.

"Okay Nancy, lean your chair back and relax. I'll be back in fifteen minutes."

By the time she returned, I was fine. I felt relaxed and ready to get the chemo. Rainey is an excellent nurse! A wonderful nurse. Overall, I've been blessed with nurses who don't insist that I "snap out of it" and follow orders. It takes great skill to read patients and respond in a way that will help them proceed.

Farewell Mr. Microphone

A few more months passed. My hair, having recovered from the Topotecan, had almost completely grown back in. Spring had arrived and the beautiful rhododendron blossoms were in their usual West Virginia splendor. I felt pretty good. Dave and I even began to plan a small summer vacation to Charleston, South Carolina, to visit Greg and Jill. We looked forward to a bit of travel now that I seemed to be stabilized and doing better.

July arrived and our blast-off for Charleston was just days away. I would get my Navelbine treatment on Friday, rest over the weekend and we'd take off on Tuesday. I went to work that Friday, planning to leave for my chemo after lunch.

It was such a gorgeous day. I remember standing outside the clinic taking in some fresh air, the warm breeze wafting past. Someone stopped to compliment me, saying I was wearing her favorite color combination: my chambray shirt and linen skirt with little blue flowers scattered across it. It was one of those brief moments your mind photographs and stores in an album with other favorite things, like the best pie you ever tasted, the smell of a clean baby, and your first glimpse of the ocean.

When I returned to my desk I felt chilled. I started to shake. I called my sister who was working at the front reception desk, "Carla, can you please go get me a hot pack? My legs are jittery. I can't warm up." I felt strange even saying the words, given that it was July in Morgantown, a valley city infamous for its sultry summers.

"What's going on?" she asked worriedly.

"I don't know. I just feel like I'm freezing to death." She thought I should leave work and I agreed, "I think I'll go home and rest and see if I start feeling better. I have chemo this afternoon."

At home I slipped into some sweats and got in bed. Just before noon I awoke, burning up! My face was flushed. I thought it was because I had on so many clothes and that I'd probably just gotten over a fever. I called the Cancer Center and asked if I should still come out for my chemo, given the circumstances. I spoke to a nurse who said she'd like for me to see the doctor first. I took her suggestion and had Dave drive me to the appointment.

When he asked me what had happened that morning I pooh-poohed the incident, "Ahh, it was nothing. I was cold at work, so I went home and got in bed to warm up and rest. I guess I must have had a fever, but it broke and I'm fine now. Just get me my chemo. I'm leaving on vacation Tuesday."

The doctor said I should skip this chemo dose. He asked me to give a urine sample so he could rule out an infection before I left for my vacation. Once on the commode I began to shake so much that I couldn't steady myself enough to pee in the cup. I didn't understand what was happening to me. The shakes suddenly got worse.

I managed to get to the door and yell down the hall for help. His physician's assistant, Renee, heard my call and ran to the rescue. I couldn't walk on my own. She somehow managed to get me to a bed and then ran to get Dave and the doctor. Dave came into the room and lay on top of me to try and stop the violent shaking.

Suddenly, I was surrounded by the medical staff. They were trying to draw blood from my port to run some quick tests. I remember my feet jutting uncontrollably up in the air. The staff kept putting their hands to my face, I guess to feel for a temperature change. I thought I was freezing to death. Then I started to vomit. There was a pull-down commode in the room and with help, I made my way to it.

The doctor stood near me and explained, "Nancy, I think you have an infection."

"No," I objected, "I have to get my chemo and I have to take my vacation."

Rainey, the attending nurse, had taken care of me in the past. She was familiar with my propensity to protest and call the shots, and my strong tendency to avoid hospitalization. To add a bit of humor to the situation she leaned down, smiling, and whispered tauntingly in my ear, "You know, you *goin'* to the big house!"

I knew she was right and reluctantly admitted it. Indeed, I *was* quite sick. This shaking episode was more violent than the others, and for the first time a fever accompanied it. The doctor had ordered an I.V. antibiotic to be administered immediately through my port, before I ever set foot out of the Cancer Center. He came by and rubbed my arm in a gesture of reassurance, "You'll be okay. You'll be all right Nancy." Someone came with a wheelchair to take me to the hospital to be admitted. It was early afternoon now and I was still throwing up. Numerous tests were being run, including X-rays to check for a sinus infection, but no news was coming.

By evening I was just lying still in my hospital bed. Around ten or eleven my blood pressure started to plummet. I knew something was up because the nurse remained at my bedside and kept the cuff on my arm. She kept asking every minute or so, "Are you okay?" "Still okay?" "You doing okay?" Even though I felt a bit out of it I kept replying that I was fine. Then she started asking me what day it was, what time it was, etc. I knew it was Friday and by looking out the window I guessed it was evening sometime.

A doctor came in from the intensive care unit and asked kindly, "Mrs. Lofstead, how are you feeling?"

I rolled onto my side to face him, and with a trace of spunk still at my disposal, I stuck both hands out and told him "I feel with my fingers." I guess it was the wrong answer because the nurse then told him I must be a bit disoriented. He explained I was headed to I.C.U., "Your blood pressure is dropping and we need to hook you up to some equipment so we can monitor you more closely." What's all the ruckus? I thought. I was ready to ask if I could submit another answer...anything to keep me out of I.C.U., but I was already on my way.

Once there, a whole squad of staff people was racing around me, hanging bags of stuff and slapping electrodes on me. Amidst all of the electronic beeping and buzzing I caught their attention when I announced I had to go to the bathroom.

Somebody came to my side with a bedpan, which I summarily rejected, explaining I'd need the real thing. The two nurses attending to me flashed the collective look of a mom who's just bundled her kid in a cumbersome ten-buckle snowsuit, only to momentarily pose the question, "Why didn't you say so before????" They started unhooking and unstrapping all these contraptions and I made my way across the room to another one of those handy-dandy pull-down commodes.

The seriousness of my condition began to sink in when someone told me my blood pressure had fallen to around 60 over 30. Records confirm my systolic pressure (120 in a healthy person) was just 70 at the time I was moved to I.C.U. They were administering a drug called dopamine. I resided there in Intensive Care for the next day and a half, not knowing if I was dying or just exactly what was happening to me—only that the road to South Carolina now had a formidable detour.

When Dave arrived at my room the next morning he was scared to death by the complex scene. He'd been phoned around midnight and told I was in I.C.U. but stable and there was no need for him to come in. I'd felt scared and was a little upset that Dave wasn't there when everything transpired, but he was just going by what the staff had told him. Along with Dave, my mom and dad soon arrived, and then Carla. They, too, were very concerned by what greeted them.

It seemed none of them understood my exact condition. When I asked Carla to help me use the bathroom and I started heading toward the corner of the room where the pull-down commode was discreetly stowed, she thought I was delirious and disoriented and kept trying to redirect me to a restroom down the hall. (Many I.C.U. patients have a urinary catheter, so those rooms aren't usually outfitted with a full bathroom.)

I was finally moved back to a regular room where I stayed for three or four days, dealing with the news of something called "septic shock"—an infection in my port line. There was no sign of infection on the skin, so it was a tricky diagnosis. I thanked God that the problem had resolved itself in Morgantown, under the care of my own doctor. Had the symptoms occurred away from home I might have died!

The port would have to be removed. This came as quite a surprise, given that my little "microphone" and I had been together for three years! Typically ports don't last that long, especially if the patient is the one doing the dressing changes, but I'd been diligent in caring for it. Concerned about how I'd get my chemo, I was told a new port would go in after a course of antibiotics was fed (round-the-clock) through the existing line during my recuperation at home. The antibiotic was prepackaged in small plastic bottles that I had to feed into the port every eight hours.

By the time I returned home from the hospital I'd lost a lot of weight. Dave phoned Judy in Cleveland, "Your mission, Judy, should you decide to accept it, is to come to West Virginia and fatten up Nancy!" She accepted. The next day she and her husband Jim showed up and started cooking and helping me with the antibiotics.

Two weeks after finishing the antibiotic, Dad took me to the hospital. I'd been told to report to the E.R. to have my "microphone" removed. There a doctor numbed my chest and pulled the line out, causing an internal tickling sensation as he did so. Even though the procedure was very painful, I wanted to see the thing that had fed me chemo for the past three years. The doctor kept trying to turn my head away, but I persisted. "Hey, you're not going to cut it, are you?" I asked. "I want that! It's a nice little necklace!" He obliged me and handed over my hard-won souvenir.

While it was a great feeling to be able to shower without the usual concern over getting the port site wet, I felt my lifeline had been severed. I felt sort of naked without the little tubes dangling from their anchorage in my bosom.

A Pint of Vertigo

Not long after I finished the antibiotic and had the port removed, another puzzling saga arose. One day I simply stood up to walk down the hall and found I couldn't manage it. I was wobbling all over! "Oh my God, Dave! Something's wrong! I'm so dizzy I can't walk," I yelled. He immediately drove me to the E.R.

The attending doctor wanted a list of my symptoms. I could only tell him that I was dizzy and unable to walk. I listed the three drugs I'd taken in the hospital during my run-in with the septic shock: Mefoxin, Gentamicin, and dopamine. There didn't seem to be any reasonable explanation for the problem.

"Nancy, I know you don't want to hear this, but I think we need to look for a tumor in your brain," he explained regretfully.

"I don't think you're going to find one, but if you insist, then I'll go ahead with it," I said. We did a lot of praying as I prepared for the M.R.I. God blessed me once again. The tests came back showing there was no brain tumor to contend with. We were all relieved, but still anxious for an explanation for my condition.

I had to hold on to the walls just to make it through the house. I simply could not function. I certainly couldn't drive. The dizzy sensation continued, seemingly a permanent addition to the list of ailments competing for my attention.

During a visit to my primary care physician she casually asked what had been going on with me. When I told her about the dizziness and listed the drugs I'd been given in July, she seemed puzzled, "Why rule out the Gentamicin? It's infamous for causing otoxicity or vertigo." The mystery was solved. An overlooked clue provided the answer. I was disappointed at the delayed diagnosis. I'd endured so many unnecessary trials—sleeping with a weird collar on while sitting up, among other tests of equilibrium.

The good news was finally finding the villain. The bad news: there would be no justice! There's nothing that can be done to reverse the vertigo. At times it nauseated me. I couldn't even ride in the car without staring straight at the floor or ceiling to avoid getting ill. It appeared to me that the car was swerving all over the road and any objects in sight seemed to jump out of place. It would be mid-September before I could return to work, but even then I had to carpool with my neighbor Linda. It was January before I could manage being behind the wheel.

There are still some lingering effects of the condition. Even today I can't go in a dark room. My balance is so bad that I have trouble with the shadows. If I walk down a street where the trees are casting intermittent shadows I lose my balance—I look like I'm drunk as I try to walk.

One weekend that September Greg and Jill came to town from South Carolina for a West Virginia football game. I was eager to get out and have some fun but I told my son he'd have to help me down into the stands to our seats, "I'll probably even have to hold on to you."

"That's okay Mom, we'll get you there in one piece," he reassured me.

I felt like I kept bumping into people along the route to our seat, so I was continually apologizing, "Excuse me. Excuse me. Sorry. I have vertigo. Sorry."

Suddenly a guy slapped me on the back and announced, "Oh, thhhhat'sss okay honey, I'm drunk myself."

"No, no, you don't understand," I explained fervently, "I have vertigo!"

But it was clear from his dazed expression he'd be looking for a pint of the stuff during his next trip to the liquor store.

Having My Pick

By now summer was nearing its end and the pulse of our college town had pumped back to life. Like many traditions, the perennial sights provided a degree of comfort given my late summer's otherwise chaotic and unpredictable sequence of events. At the Dairy Queen near campus the lines of customers extending from the two windows now wrapped down the street like a pair of braids. The extra traffic meant leaving a few minutes earlier for work. The aisles at Wal-Mart were filled with co-eds buying laundry baskets, shower curtains, and discounted toasters—the stuff kids take for granted until it's their turn to outfit a home.

That old familiar panic was settling in over the fact that there was no chemo going into my body and the tumors could be starting to grow again. My Baltimore oncologist asked me to come out and have what's called a "PIC line" inserted into my left arm. PIC stands for peripherally inserted catheter.

With my arm under a fluoroscope, the tiny line was fed up into the vein from just below the elbow. It went all the way up to the shoulder and into the "superior vena cava"—the driveway to my heart! As part of the line upkeep the PIC had to be flushed daily with both saline and Heparin solutions using needle-less syringes. That was Dave's job. I didn't like the line being in my arm, but I did like the little cap on the end because it was similar to the one on my beloved Hickman.

The PIC would serve as my temporary host for chemo infusions. It fascinated me to know that medications administered through the PIC would reach the heart within eight seconds of entering my arm. Once I was healed and fully recovered from the septic shock another "permanent" port would go into place.

I was very active—not the "typical cancer patient," the medical folks were always telling me. The line tended to slip out a bit here and there. I'd hang quilts out on the clothesline on the weekend. Slip. I'd play around with our dog Winston. Slip. Eventually I'd be forced to place the call to Baltimore, "Uhm. Well, um, it seems to have come out about another quarter inch or so..."

"Nancy, WHAT have you been doing?" the nurse would question.

Expert in the art of playing dumb, I'd apologize, "I can't help it. It seems to have just pulled out a bit more."

Soon the little cap that was at mid-forearm on the day the line was inserted had meandered down to my wrist. I recall sitting in a meeting or two where I'd lost track of its placement.

"What on earth is hanging out of your sleeve?" some naïve soul would ask.

Without explanation, I'd pick up the tiny device and speak into it, "Testing one-two-three, testing one-two-three."

I had a blast with it for around seven weeks, about the maximum length of time the temporary line is usually left in. During that stretch, though, I'd pester the staff in Baltimore. "I want this thing out of my arm. I hate it. It's too uncomfortable," I'd complain. I was asked to schedule an appointment for October so that I could have the PIC removed and a new "porta-cath" installed in my chest.

When the PIC was removed I saw that the line was much longer than I'd envisioned—why had I worried over a couple inches slipping out here and there? I didn't understand what all the panic had been about, the thing was nearly long enough to use as a jump rope!

"This new one will be under your skin," the doctor explained to me. A special "Huber" needle would be used to access the porta-cath to administer the chemo.

Hmmm...*under* the skin? The image triggered an idea for a little prank I decided to pull on the doctor. I bought a seven-inch-long zipper and took it with me to the hospital. Dave knew about the scheme and so did the anesthesiologist.

"Okay, I'm going to need your help with this," I plotted. "I'm going to tape this zipper to my chest where the port is supposed to go so the doctor gets a little chuckle when he begins the procedure. You with me? Your job is to conceal it while I'm being put under so the surprise is preserved, got it?" He got it. He laughed. He was a willing accomplice if I ever saw one.

The time came for me to enter the O.R. My doctor, along with the anesthesiologist, the nurse and nurse's assistant, approached. He asked jovially, "Are you ready? Let's get going." Off we marched like a team of scouts. I felt especially devilish.

On the way we passed a little lady stationed at a counter. "Would you like a hot blanket?" she asked sweetly.

"How much are they today?" I inquired.

"Ten thenth," she lisped.

"Okay, I'll take two." I turned to look at the doctor and his staff, "Anybody back there want a hot blanket? They're only ten cents." Nobody took me up on the offer.

In the O.R. I was surrounded by people wearing serious faces and big plastic surgical shields. They were busily sorting out the instruments for use in my procedure. "HEY, how's everybody doing today?" I said, announcing my presence like a comedian warming up a crowd for the big act to follow. I continued, "What are you guys doing?"

My doctor was getting that pre-exasperation look, "No jokes today, okay Nancy? You're not getting ready to tell a joke, are you?"

"Well, no, actually, I wasn't," I replied innocently, "Besides, I think when I start to tell a joke in here you give a nod to the guy behind me who puts me out before I ever get to finish it anyway."

"No I don't," he denied.

"Yes you do. I don't remember ever finishing one of my jokes when I'm in your O.R."

"Go ahead," he said, indulging me.

"Well," I began, mustering all the sincerity of a nun raising money for orphans, "I just want to tell you I'm convinced there will be a medical breakthrough here today! What is about to be performed here has never occurred in any other operating room anywhere at any time!"

"Okay, Okay, Nancy," sighed my doctor, "I need your arm out of the gown." I looked at the anesthesiologist thinking, okay buddy, this is where you have to help me. And he did.

I woke up in recovery and began my usual process of tap-tap-tapping—just to be sure someone's aware I'm alive and starting to wake up. *I'm* always afraid they won't remember I'm there and *they* always tell me not to tap with the little plastic blood oxygen monitor strapped to my finger. They say the tapping damages it. "Just wanted you to know I'm awake," I announced.

"Okay! We know you're awake," came the reply as if from across a wide river.

I looked up at a clock and thought, hey, that little process didn't last too long. I felt just a tad cocky, telling myself, "I have my new port in. Any minute now someone should be wheeling me to the Cancer Center for my dose of Navelbine and to be sure the port's working." Something seemed strange. Everyone who walked by smiled and waved. Some laughed. I joined many of them in conversations I was not meant to be a part of.

I kept hearing the nurses asking, "Where are Betty and Sue?"

Someone would answer, "They went to lunch."

I piped up, "Would you like me to page them? I can get on the intercom and page them, no problem." I was an experienced pager from my years of working at the physical therapy clinic.

"No thanks, we're okay, you just rest."

"You let me know if I should page them, okay?" I loudly volunteered again. I don't know where this stuff was coming from, I just felt particularly talkative coming out of the anesthesia. The nurses had to be thinking, somebody give that lady something to shut her up!

At one point I innocently reached up to scratch my forehead. Then I knew why everyone was laughing and smiling. The doctor had dealt his touché! Taped to my forehead was the seven-inch-long pink zipper I'd last seen adhered to my chest just before surgery! It's true what they say about paybacks!

Eventually I was wheeled over to Outpatient for my chemo. There I met a nurse who'd taken care of me three years earlier, back in 1994. It was great seeing her again and we spent a lot of time chatting. I told her about the little convertible I'd bought since we were last in contact, "We drove it up here today. Tell you what, when we leave here in a minute, I'll have Dave drive a lap up here by the window so you can all see it." They jokingly told me I'd have to stand up and wave as we passed.

Sooner or later people who know me learn they shouldn't unthinkingly toss out dares. Despite having just undergone the surgery to install the porta-cath in my chest, and just finishing the Navelbine infusion, I stood proudly on the seat of the car. I waved wildly at my old friend and her co-workers, who waved back, each of them wearing a look that clearly said, "That woman is truly mad!"

I loved having this particular port. It's totally under the skin so I don't have to shower with caution. It's accessed by needle only when necessary. I continued my Navelbine treatments here at the Cancer Center in Morgantown.

For Better, For Worse, In Sickness and In Health

This year Dave and I celebrated our 32nd wedding anniversary...an event that seemed impossible to imagine back in 1969, when we'd said "I do" not long after leaving high school and barely prepared to maintain an apartment or a car, much less a marriage, but we were so much in love. And maintain is exactly what we've done over the past three decades—me and the guy I long ago nicknamed "Bumstead."

Dave is my rock. To me, his tall, square frame seems as strong as it was in the old days when he was a high school basketball star and I was on the sidelines in my cheerleader uniform and bobby socks. At practice he'd cruise up near me, grinning and whispering in my ear, "You know you love me. You *know* you love me, why not just admit it?" Instinctively, with the same confidence that scored basket after basket for our team, Dave knew I was the one for him. The conclusion was somewhat less obvious to me at first.

Dave and I started dating just before our junior year at University High. One reason I felt attracted to him was because of his wit. I had classes with Dave and saw the jokester in action. I remember one time in our political science class the teacher asked him why his homework was missing. Without skipping a beat, this teenager who would later become my betrothed stood up and humbly explained that his mother was in jail. "Now, I don't want anyone feeling sorry for my twin brother Danny and me, but we've had it pretty rough at home because of Mom's situation," he improvised. He kept the teachers and students laughing. It was hard not to like the guy!

For Dave, having a twin brother meant sharing a car. Sharing a car meant guaranteeing transportation for our dates was impossible! The '56 Chevy the boys drove at the time was the object of more than one brotherly tug-of-war. Given that my family lived outside of town near the lake, it wasn't like he could just pop over and walk me to the movies.

My parents weren't too thrilled with this guy who'd call to cancel plans at the last minute because his wheels had suddenly disappeared, at least not in the beginning. Eventually Dave buffaloed my mom into always taking his side when he and I would have one of the little spats or temporary break-ups that dotted our high school romance.

He was not the kind of guy to dress up or get excited about formal dances and that sort of thing, even though *I* wanted to go. Then why did it upset him so much when one of his basketball buddies asked me to the prom and I accepted? I remember being out on the dance floor in my stunning Sixties gown—pale green with embroidered daisies on the bodice, empire waist, huge bow on the back, my hair piled up on top of my head. But wait, is someone cutting in? I'm feeling a distinct tug on the back of my dress.

Guess who? Yep! Standing there in his letter jacket and blue jeans, Dave was practically demanding that I leave the dance with him. I refused and reminded him that he didn't want to be at the prom in the first place but *I* did! His next move was to follow my date and me back to my place. He waited until the other guy left and then came in the house for a long chat with my mother. Together they mulled over the one big question he grappled with, "Doesn't she understand that *I'm* the one who should be with her?"

Apparently I didn't. The next year I went to the prom with yet another guy. Forget his athletic prowess, Dave still doesn't like to dance. He can be talked into the occasional slow dance and that's about it. But then, dancing's not everything. Despite our little falling-outs, I knew the two of us had a neat bond. Dave was just much more casual, and more of a homebody than I. I'm the one who's rambunctious, who wants to rip into the Christmas gifts early. Dave's the methodical one who makes me wait until the prescribed hour to open the presents.

I remember how much he hated having his classmates choose him as king of the May Court. *I* was a queen candidate but lost out to a beautiful girl who'd also (!!) beaten me out in the vote for homecoming queen. That meant changing the line-up of escorts just before the grand march. Poor Dave was flustered by this chain of events and absolutely couldn't stand wearing that goofy little crown on his head! It was the price he paid for being popular! Everybody liked the Lofstead twins. In fact, Danny had been "king" material at homecoming time, and might have worn his own crown if he hadn't been caught spreading lime on the football field at Morgantown High (our arch rivals) and rendered ineligible for the court!

When Dave was named to the conference All-Star basketball team our senior year, yours truly was the cheerleader picked to cheer at the big game. It was an exciting time for the two of us. By then, I knew the big blonde ballplayer with the quirky sense of humor had a point when I'd hear him whisper, "You know you love me, don't you?"

The love that began way back then has sustained us through the years. We'd both started college in the fall after high school. Dave went to Fairmont State and I went to WVU. We were both intending to major in phys ed, but those plans were set aside in our freshman year when our major switched to parenthood! We married in January of 1969. That summer Greg entered the world to the ecstatic greetings of his father, who was already picturing the kid shooting lay-ups and mastering the spiral pass, among a host of other sports moves.

This proud papa, not even old enough to vote at the time, took on the responsibility like a man twice his age. As a student he'd "worked" part-time delivering furniture and appliances for a local store along with his buddy. Unbeknownst to their boss and the customers, between stops these two seasoned professionals gave the truck a rest and enjoyed long layovers for cokes and pinball games. Those lazy days did a rapid vanishing act when he became a husband and father-to-be.

My mom and dad's neighbor knew Dave was looking for a real job and suggested Dave join him working at a company called Weston Chemicals (now General Electric). He has worked there ever since and is now among the three or four most senior employees at the Morgantown plant, having worked his way up to a management position.

Dave's been the perfect provider—always intent on making sure we had what we needed. I was able to stay home and care for Greg, and then for Geoff, who was born three and a half years later.

Over time we have watched other married couples spend carefree years together and develop their careers before starting a family. We'd always pictured our marriage in reverse: first raise a family and then have our "just the two of us" leisure time. Cancer drastically changed that picture for us. By the time the boys were raised we were hobnobbing to hospitals and chemo treatments instead of romantic resorts.

It goes to show you that it doesn't help to plan life out too far in advance. We were such young parents; we practically grew up along with our sons. I don't regret that at all. Dave and I had fun raising them. We spent a lot of time with them because we were just kids ourselves. This is a life we've built year by year.

Through it all Dave's been a pillar of strength for me. He's always saying, "Honey, put on your boxing gloves. You gotta get right back up and fight this thing that's trying to knock you out!" Now *he's* on the sidelines cheering and I'm in there giving it my all. When I've tried to get him to discuss preparations in the event of a T.K.O., he won't hear of it. Dave is not the type to plan for the worst outcome while there's still hope for the best.

"For better, for worse, in sickness and in health…" If any couple has thought about the words that make up those stock wedding vows, we sure have.

How many other husbands would patiently stand by in the baby food aisle of the grocery store while their wife deliberates over her supper menu? And in my book, no meal is complete without dessert. I remember us getting a few stares from other shoppers when Dave asked, "Okay Honey, decide. Which sounds better tonight, a jar of blueberry buckle or peach cobbler?" Cancer forces people to write new definitions for terms like "supper," "ordinary life," "the future," and "marriage."

As the months and years have passed in my battle with this relentless disease, Dave has been there, helping me to redefine these things and other stuff healthy folks routinely take for granted. He can be the tough guy or he can sit and cry right along with me. The other day I said, "Honey, I'm so sorry you're having to go through this."

He looked at me and shook his head, "Wait a minute. Just wait a minute. What if the tables were turned? What if it were *me* with cancer?" When I told him I'd be right there for him he said, "That's what I mean. Don't ever say you're sorry about the illness."

I guess it's my feeling of dependence. It can become almost overwhelming at times and make me feel apologetic. But I should know better. He's the one to say, "Go ahead and rest after work. I'll make a nice dinner when I get home." We'd already been through enough together, enduring some pretty tough times, that when the cancer came along, we felt we could certainly weather this storm.

At one point I went from my chemo treatment to the beauty shop and asked our stylist to neatly buzz my hair all off, saying, "Leave just a bit more on top than Dave has." Shortly after that, I drove home from work one day and was coming up the steps from the garage when I heard him say, "Close your eyes Honey, I've got a surprise for you!" I sensed he'd shaved his head and I was right!

"I kinda like this!" he said, running his hand over the stubble and implying he'd gotten the cut in a gesture of solidarity.

"Hey, that's no sacrifice," I teased him, "You didn't have much hair to begin with. Why didn't you do it earlier, when you still had something to cut?"

Dave still shaves his head—somewhat out of necessity. It never fully grew back after his little surprise. I've overheard him tell people, "It's not fair. Nancy's lost her hair four times and it's always grown back in. I lost mine once and it's still gone!"

Hair or no hair, Dave's my better half. "This is just a bend in the road," he'll tell me, "We're going to go through some more bends before we get on the straight path again." I can't imagine not having this intimacy to nurture me along throughout the journey. I don't know what I would do without my best friend at my side to fight this disease...the guy who used to sidle up to me in his basketball shoes, cocky and smirking, "You *know* you love me, don't you?"

CHAPTER 5

A Celebration Called Life

1997- 2000

Cancer with an Attitude

Sometimes it's not a close friend or relative whose support reaches down into the soul of a survivor. Sometimes it's a stranger. Someone who's been there and lived to tell about it. I've found that a major part of my journey with cancer involves helping others travel along their own path. It wasn't anything I planned. My advocacy has evolved as naturally as the slope of a West Virginia horizon.

Oftentimes throughout the years the same oncology nurses who cared for me way back in '89 during my first inpatient chemo treatments right after diagnosis, would telephone and ask for my help. "Nancy, could you please come over to the hospital? We've got a patient who's really struggling. Someone who needs to see you." I assured them they were welcome to call me and that I'd be glad to help wherever I could. I'd pop over to the hospital on my lunch break to meet the patient they were concerned about.

One day a nurse called and asked that I come to meet an ovarian cancer patient named Jane who was really having a hard time. I agreed and told her I'd be there around noon. A second call soon came, "Nancy, can you please come NOW?" I explained that I was busy at work and couldn't get away until lunchtime. The nurse pleaded, "You have to come now. She's being discharged. She's having a *very* tough time. She needs to see you!" I relented, made a hasty explanation to my co-workers, and headed out the door, bound for the oncology department.

I walked into the woman's hospital room and with one quick glance, spotted the familiar badge of a chemo patient. She'd lost all of her hair, save for the few straggly threads that dotted her scalp. I introduced myself, "Hi. I'm Nancy Lofstead. I have ovarian cancer. I came to—"

The woman leapt toward me and threw her arms around my shoulders, nearly causing us to fall and almost knock a picture off the wall in the process. Her excitement would not be contained, "YOU have cancer?! You look so normal!" She grabbed my hand and quickly made a close inspection, "You have nails! They're polished! You're wearing make-up...you look so, so normal. You're dressed up!"

"Of course I'm normal," I responded, feeling a bit like a very human-looking alien at the hands of a bewildered astronomer.

"Will I be like this, too?" she asked hopefully.

I assured her she would. Hair grows back. Attitude returns. We survivors know how to work it. Fortunately she's never had a recurrence.

Jane is still my friend. I'd stop by the hospital for visits while she sat through her chemo treatments. A couple other women getting their chemo would join us. We'd talk and laugh, carrying on so loudly we were asked to move to the solarium and keep it down. There's a special bond among the members of this particular "women's club."

Today she lives in Georgia so we keep in touch with email and phone calls. It's not like the old days when she lived in a nearby town and we'd meet for dessert at a local restaurant to catch up. I even met Jane's parents when she brought them to my house for a visit. Jane is among the precious friends I call my "cancer cousins"— those people I've come to know and love through the common bond of our shared illness.

There's not much hesitation on my part when it comes to meeting with someone who needs me. Like Jane, a lot of cancer patients need a positive image of the future so they have something to shoot for. Speaking from experience, it's unfamiliar territory when you're first diagnosed and being there on your own makes navigation pretty scary.

If I find myself questioning whether or not to get involved and counsel a particular patient, I simply ask the question, "What would God want me to do?" Then the answer is simple. He's never turned his back on me. *I* couldn't turn away from someone who's sick. Someone who is saying, "I need your help."

It's true that over the last dozen years Dave has often born the brunt of my outreach to so many cancer patients. It can mean spending time away from home or hours on the phone. It can be mentally and emotionally exhausting. I've had many close friends say, "Now remember Nancy, you're Number One. You have to take care of yourself first."

That approach didn't cut it for me. I'd reason, "What if the people *I* need were to turn away?"

I think if there's no one there to support those patients, they won't believe they can make it through. I try to put myself in their shoes. Besides, looking back, it's clear they've ministered to me as much as I have to them. The frequent emotional drain that comes from supporting someone through treatment can be difficult, yet I get so much out of that very personal, meaningful experience.

At times, when the demand for my stamina seemed extreme, I'd remind myself of my strong belief that God doesn't give us more of a burden than we can carry. However, sometimes I do question His assessment of me—maybe God thinks I'm a stronger person than I really am?! Maybe I need to tell Him, "Excuse me, I'm not quite that strong...you can ease up any time now."

There were times I probably didn't return patient phone calls as soon as I should have. I may have been battling my own exhaustion at the same time they needed me to help them cope with theirs. But God knows when we can take it. My mother was always there to listen. She'd say, "We'll pray about it." The "it" could be my cancer or any other challenge I was trying to deal with. I'm convinced that helping others has been a key to my own survival.

Being a support has brought me in touch with so many wonderful people I would otherwise never have met. The cancer connected us. Like Jane. She's told me many times that she's tried to pass on the gift I gave her back when she was fighting cancer. She's not afraid to say the words, "I'm a cancer survivor." She understands the importance of a good support system and she knows the great feeling that comes from directing your own care. She's called more than once to say, "Hey, I pulled a 'Nancy' today!"

Then she'd elaborate, "I told the doctor I was leaving town, even after he informed me I couldn't go!" She then described a situation where the doctor tried to talk her into staying put, but ultimately caved in to her unwavering determination, insisting she'd have to get her labs taken and not leave town if her counts were down. Jane and her husband drove their camper straight to the hospital where she stubbornly proclaimed, "I'm sitting here until the labs come back, because I *am* leaving town!" I feel just a twinge of admiration for my little cancer-fighting protégé.

When the people I've worked with take it upon themselves to help others, there's a succession of caring in place. It's also teaching by example. If I take charge of my medical care, and have at least some say in the direction of my treatment, then surely they can too. It helps the rookie patient to work from a cancer cousin's example.

I see my work as having a ripple effect, even though not everyone is cut out to wave a banner and march down Main Street in the cancer survivor parade. Some folks are extremely private. I spoke frankly with a woman who'd had breast cancer years ago. She told me she felt guilty about not carrying on the kind of work I was doing, the effort that put us in touch with each other.

"Why feel guilty?" I asked.

"Because you have given to so many people," she explained.

I tried to comfort her with one very basic fact, "But you have given silently without even knowing it."

I was sure of this, given her active membership in "Reach to Recovery," a breast cancer survivor group. I told her that we all give in our own way, and that not everyone is comfortable or even capable of serving as an individual support network. I've had others say, "I wish I could do what you do, but I can't." Some folks want to close the chapter of life that covers their fight with cancer and never look back. That's okay. It's such an individual thing; you just can't be judgmental about that choice.

⚘

I am often reminded of those patients I met who were extremely secretive about their illness. Many times only a few close relatives or friends were even aware of their cancer. Their intense desire for privacy is another one of those highly personal issues with no right or wrong stance.

Several years after I learned I had cancer, the gynecologist who diagnosed me called to ask if I'd go visit a patient who'd just found out she had ovarian cancer. I can vividly recall walking into her hospital room and introducing myself. We made small talk but she never mentioned the word "cancer." It was as if not speaking the word would make the condition disappear.

When I said good-bye, her husband cornered me in the hospital corridor, gesturing with a stack of papers he'd brought from the library. "Look at this," he said sternly, "According to this she's not going to live long. It's true, isn't it?"

"Throw it away!" I suggested. "Those are statistics. They're based on all sorts of factors. They mean nothing. She's alive, isn't she? Start with that."

I sent her cards and notes of encouragement. I continued to visit the woman as she received her chemo treatments. I was amazed at how she'd turned a simple hospital room into a command post for their family business. There was a fax machine at her bedside. She'd brought her own colorful, flowered comforter and pillows from home. It was as if she'd merely set up a branch office in the oncology ward instead of checking in as a seriously ill patient. She's still alive today.

For me, it's been important to let people know it's possible to survive and that it's okay to be vocal about the struggle. Unlike the woman who couldn't (or wouldn't) discuss her disease, my choice is to talk out loud about cancer, rather than speak in the hushed tones of my grandmother's era. It's how I go about educating the people I come in contact with.

This is not the type of conversation every cancer survivor is willing to have, opening up to a total stranger and sharing the intimate details of one's menacing encounter(s) with the "Big C." Personally, I feel a strong need to speak out. The more people know about this disease the better they'll be able to fight it. Maybe the education we provide for each other, and the comfort we can offer in sharing our own experiences, will help someone else survive.

I recently overheard a man attempting a sort of "explanation" for his wife's diminished health. Instead of speaking in a normal tone, he whispered apologetically, "She has *breast cancer.*"

In my view, survival means confronting cancer. It means talking out loud, without the shame implied by shadowy tones and whispers like the ones that floated just out of earshot of my poor Aunt Emma in the months preceding her death. It means drawing courage from our very humanness, the two-sided coin that, should we choose to give it a flip, can just as easily define us as weak and sickly.

I've had people tell me they've never been around someone who could make them laugh about cancer, or just laugh in general, when they're ill or hurting. I think laughter is an important key to survival, right up there with good doctors and effective, tolerable medicine. Laughter offers its own component to the healing process, but a lot of people can't move out of the dreary shadow cancer likes to cast.

I'm reminded of a conversation with a man who had just joined our clinic staff, back at the time I was wearing my wig. He approached me one day in a polite manner and asked if we could talk. As a courtesy, he wanted to acknowledge that he knew about the cancer and ask how I was handling things. After a pause, he said, "And if you don't mind my asking, how does it feel to wear that wig?"

"To tell you the truth, it feels like a UFO landed on my head," I answered.

"Oh, gosh. Now there, I've gone and upset you," he said apologetically.

I reassured him, "No, no I'm not upset. I'm just kidding."

Hesitantly, he continued his line of questioning about the wig, "How do you keep it on?"

"Simple," I began. "In the front I use a staple gun and in the back I pound in a few carpet tacks."

"Oh now I've REALLY upset you, I'm sorry. I'm so sorry," he stammered, backing away in retreat. I let him know I was just having some fun—that it's one of the ways I cope with my situation.

Lots of books make the point about laughter, along with the importance of sharing. I'm not embarrassed for anyone to know I have cancer, so I share my story and whatever information they care to know. Opening myself up to others releases some of the burden from within.

It's amazing what you can find out about a person sitting next to you in a room filled with strangers. If a show of hands were asked for, there might be twenty people in that room who've been touched by cancer. These days it's hard to find someone whose life *hasn't* been affected by the disease—an unfortunate common denominator in our time!

⸎

When I try to educate cancer patients about some of the elements of survival, I always emphasize my deep belief in the benefit of letting go of past suffering, "You're going to need all your energy to focus on recovering." Holding on to past hurts and disappointments uses up precious emotional and spiritual resources that could be enlisted in the fight for survival. I've talked to many patients who want desperately to blame somebody.

It's always, "If my doctor had only done this or that…" or "If only someone had told me sooner that…"

No matter WHAT has happened, the truth is, the bad stuff from the past is heavy baggage for anyone to carry, much less someone battling a life-threatening illness. I tell them to move forward. You can't heal with negativity. You have to be positive to successfully walk down the steep, muddy path of cancer survival.

My hope is that people who witness my outlook will think, "Hey it seems to be working for her. I'll have what she's having." Yet I don't expect them to come back to me and say, "Because *you* did this or that, I did too." I would just like to know I've had some helpful effect on the patients I've tried to reach, accepting the fact that we're all different and eventually everyone will react in his or her own way.

I continue to be asked about my strong beliefs regarding cancer survival. I'm still singing the same tune after all these years. Much of my approach centers on my faith in God and prayer. It's part of my time-tested theory that attitude accounts for at least 80% of the reason some of us beat the odds...always with the assumption that there's a backdrop of good medical care, which means a doctor/patient "team" approach. I don't want to downplay the physician's role in beating cancer, or the chemotherapy, or whatever treatment is prescribed, but I think the right attitude is crucial.

If you don't believe in your ability to fight it, to deal with whatever comes along, you're contributing to your own downfall. Back when I was fainting due to the exertion I felt when just trying to get through my own house, I forced myself to crawl. I thought if I stopped in my tracks I was surrendering my body to cancer, an act I refused to carry out.

This whole thing is one big arm wrestle, but an arm wrestle you don't have to handle alone. If cancer patients can find a doctor who's willing to work with them, then they're allowed to say, "This is *my* life. This is what *I* want. This is how *I* will deal with cancer." It's very empowering. My doctor understands this mandate in my treatment.

He might write up a list of chemo drugs that I could potentially take and I'll give it the once-over. I'm not afraid to let him hear my layperson's conclusions, "Nope, can't do this one. It would really cramp my lifestyle. Can't do that one either. This one over here looks okay." It's as if the two of us are playing the part of car salesman and buyer. "Okay, I like the standard options on this one, but I'd never drive this color, can we order it in blue?"

As I think about it, maybe survival is *more* than 80% attitude, maybe it nearly all depends on attitude. Attitude and faith. I have tremendous faith, but I'm also a realist. I don't think I'll be around forever. I'm not that naïve.

New Year's Rockin' Eve

On New Year's Eve, Dave and I were sitting at home, planning a very low-key welcome to 1998. I'd had my usual Friday afternoon Navelbine treatment at the Cancer Center during the day and just wanted to relax and rest that night. We'd rented a few videos and settled into our nest for an uneventful evening.

Dave was enjoying sitting in the big recliner I'd bought him as a Christmas present. It had a built-in heat and massage mechanism and was really comfortable. When I saw Dave get up to do something, I made a quick move to steal the seat from him. We ended up having a disastrous game of musical chairs. As both of us headed for the coveted recliner at the same time, I launched myself into it with the determination of a base runner sliding into home plate at a World Series game. My rear landed on the back of the chair and the big recliner did a flip—with me in it!

"That's what you get for trying to steal my chair!" he joked, then added, "You *are* okay, aren't you?" I assured him everything was fine and we had a good laugh.

But on the first day of the new year I awoke to find that a small lump had formed in my chest, just above the port site and near my underarm. There was a bit of pain and the area seemed somewhat warm to me. Dave wanted to take me to the emergency room but I disagreed, "I don't want to spend my holiday afternoon crammed into a waiting room with a bunch of kids with strep throat and people who twisted their ankle in a New Year's Eve stupor."

He suggested we call my doctor in Baltimore. I didn't want to interrupt his holiday with my problem, which I told myself was probably nothing more than a little pulled muscle resulting from the chair incident. "Let's call him on Monday," I offered in a compromise. And I did just that, explaining that, no, I hadn't been drinking, and yes, I did get my Friday chemo as scheduled.

He advised me to go get a Doppler ultrasound of the upper extremities, and to have the doctor check the area under my arm and near the port site. "You could have a blood clot, Nancy," he informed me. Within minutes I was on the phone trying to reach the doctor who'd implanted my first port, the Hickman, because I'd been told he was one local physician sure to have the Doppler. The staff person told me to come right over for the ultrasound. I left work to drive to his office, telling my co-workers, "I'll be back in about an hour."

The technician applied the gel and began to check things out. She kept traveling up my neck, despite my professional opinion that she should check near the armpit, closer to the lump. "It's down here. Can't you feel it?" I said, trying to redirect her.

"Nancy, have you been having any other problems?" she asked, seeming to ignore my suggestion.

"No, I'm fine and dandy. The lump just appeared Saturday morning."

"You'd better speak with your doctor," she informed me. Then, as if to convince the "inconvincible" that something was wrong, she pointed to the monitor screen and showed me how the blood flow had drastically decreased by comparing the left side to the right. Next I learned my jugular was almost entirely occluded!

I'd had no headache, no other symptoms. The seriousness of the situation had yet to hit me. I thought, oh well, they'll give me a little Heparin or Coumadin—both are blood thinners. No big deal. Then she told me to get dressed and she left the room, returning in a moment to say my primary care doctor was on the phone.

"Nancy, how did you get to their office?" my doctor probed.

"I drove."

"I want you to get to the hospital right away," she instructed me, "I'll meet you there."

As always, I had to exercise my bargaining power, "Is that really necessary? Can't you just give me a bit of Coumadin and send me on my way?"

I could hear the nurses laughing at this suggestion from Dr. Nancy. Upon reflection, I'm sure they were appalled that I was pooh-poohing an occluded jugular.

My doctor didn't budge, "I'll meet you at the hospital! You need to get going on some Heparin. It slows the clotting time."

"Okay, okay," I acquiesced, and then borrowed the phone again to call Carla back at our office. "Carla, can you believe this? They're sending me to the hospital. There's evidently some sort of clot in the vein in my neck. I'm supposed to get over there right now." I drove to the hospital and found Carla already waiting in the lobby.

I started feeling a bit nervous. I hate not knowing what's happening to me and not being in charge. Why can't I just call the shots and forget about all this medical mumbo-jumbo? I went through registration, thinking all the while, I feel fine. I just don't understand what's going on here. The uncertainty of all this got me quite worked up.

I was escorted to my hospital room and told to undress. Soon I was throwing up. My doctor appeared and asked me what was wrong.

"I don't know," I said.

"I'll tell you what's wrong. You're not in charge here. You've lost control," she told me. "I'll have the nurses give you something to help you get settled. Now calm down."

"I'm trying to!" I snapped. It all came out of fear. I had no idea what was happening to me and I felt incredibly scared and defensive.

I was hospitalized all week long. I took Heparin and Coumadin and endured the dreaded prepping for a CAT scan, trying my best to cope with the usual bout of severe diarrhea that came with the prep. On Thursday I underwent the scan, which covered my neck and chest. Sure enough, it revealed a well-formed clot. The little dickens had been stowing away there for some time! It had even made itself comfortable in its little abode, forming collateral veins to transport the bulk of the blood from point A to point B.

Because my chest port poses an additional risk to the blood clot situation, I have to keep taking Coumadin. I get regular blood tests. My doctor routinely monitors the situation. There's really nothing more that can be done so I try not to think about it. Besides, with the cancer there are always bigger fish to fry!

No Foolin'!

A highlight of 1998 was receiving a "Community Star Award." The local newspaper grants them to area residents who've been nominated for service to their community. I could not have been more surprised when I found out my name was among the winners! It happened in a funny way.

One morning I came in to work and was told I'd received a phone call from the publisher of the *Dominion Post* (our Morgantown daily) and that I should return the call. I said, "Why in the world would he call *me*?"

Carla overheard me say this and urged me to get in touch. I mentioned I'd get to it later when I had more time. In a short while I passed by her desk. She asked eagerly, "Well? Did you call him?"

"I'll get to it when I get to it," I told her, wondering why she was showing so much interest.

"Call him!" she insisted.

I finally did.

"Nancy, this is Dave Raese from the *Dominion Post*. I was calling to congratulate you. You've won a Community Star Award," he explained.

"You must have the wrong person," I responded, thinking of how, each year, I'd read with interest the impressive list of winners and the various reasons for their nominations. "Are you looking for my sister-in-law, *Becky* Lofstead?" I continued.

"No. I'm looking for Nancy," he said.

"Who is this?" I demanded, thinking someone might be playing an early April Fool's joke on me.

"This is Dave Raese from the *Morgantown Dominion Post*. Am I speaking to Nancy Lofstead?"

"Uh huh."

"And you *do* have cancer?" he quizzed me.

"Yes I do."

"Well, you were nominated by Carla Neely and the committee then voted for you as one of the four award winners," he explained.

I was dumbfounded. I strolled out to the reception area where Carla was working and told her the good news. She was elated that her nomination had been approved. She thought my work with cancer patients, especially supporting and encouraging folks who've just been diagnosed, made me worthy of the honor. She wrote a compelling letter to the committee to tell them about my efforts.

Word about the award spread quickly around the clinic and everyone started congratulating me. I felt truly privileged to receive the recognition. It's part of the American Institute for Public Service "Jefferson Awards" program. The awards were presented at a lovely banquet later that same month. Carla and her husband John were there, along with Dave, his twin brother Dan and his wife Becky, and my dad. (Mom would have loved to join us but she was too sick at the time.)

Knowing of my reluctance to speak in public, Carla had teased me about having to get up and give an acceptance speech. I was so nervous I decided not to eat anything at the banquet. These things are better done on an empty stomach, I reasoned, even though Carla, who would be at the podium much longer than me to explain her nomination, seemed to thoroughly enjoy her meal.

She had prepared and rehearsed a short presentation, complete with official-looking note cards, but when the time came Carla ignored the cards and spoke from the heart, delivering a flawless speech to the crowded banquet room. As she finished her remarks and introduced me, I went forward to accept the award and nervously uttered a few words of thanks.

"I appreciate this award, but I really don't think I've done anything extraordinary. Why are we here if not to help one another on our journey through life? I've always believed none of us is getting out of here alive. Often we can't repay others for the kindness they've shown us, but we can at least pass it on to someone else in need."

Of the four Community Star Award winners in this area (North-Central West Virginia), I was chosen to go on to the national banquet in Washington, DC, where I met other winners from around the country. We were treated like royalty and each presented with a beautiful, bronze Jefferson Award medallion (produced at the Franklin Mint). It bears a replica of the Seal of the United States on one side. On the other is a citation for outstanding public service and the engraved signatures of three of the program's benefactors, including that of Jacqueline Kennedy Onassis. It was such an honor and one I still feel somewhat under-qualified to have received.

When I consider getting an actual, tangible reward for my work I feel a bit awkward. The greatest rewards have been those from the cancer patients themselves, or in some cases, their relatives.

I once received a note from a man thanking Dave and me for attending his wife's funeral. How often does that happen? He went on to say how grateful he was for my phone calls and the time I spent with her, a woman I'd met at the Cancer Center. During her wake he'd hugged both Dave and me in appreciation of the support I gave her.

I'd been stunned to hear she'd passed away one Saturday, just three days after visiting her at home and meeting her husband for the first time. I recall taking her a Christmas present that day—a wooden folk art angel. It was in a gift bag, but she was too weak to open it, so I helped her. Placing it on the nightstand, I said the little angel was there to keep an eye on her. I patted her leg and she sweetly smiled up at me.

It strikes me that I may speak on the phone with a cancer patient for a year, and perhaps never meet her or her family in person, while in other cases I'm introduced shortly after a patient's diagnosis. I come in contact with so many people who have cancer. People feel the need to tell me about anyone close to them who's got cancer. Sometimes I'll hear about three new people in just a day or two. Word might come in a call from a family member I'll never meet or from a co-worker I see every day.

For a time I was sending cards to a lady I was especially concerned about. I came home from work one day, hit the message button on the answering machine, and heard her mother's voice tell me that she'd passed away. "She talked about you all the time," the mother added, bringing tears to my eyes. I wanted to go to the funeral home but I just couldn't. Another time a woman (a cancer cousin's daughter) brought me the gift of a book, something her father had asked her to do for me just before he died.

Dave thinks it would be too hard on me to attend all of the wakes and funerals, and he's right. A person can only handle so much grief, I guess. Every time I lose a cancer cousin a little piece of me rips away. It's such an emotional thing—just admitting that someone I can relate to has lost the battle. I can't help thinking that it could easily be me in their place, maybe two years down the road, or maybe in just two months.

It's been a tremendous gift to be able to minister to people who are still surviving. Their success helps give me hope and make me want to keep fighting. Sometimes I question my own example to others. Maybe my struggle with the recurrences gives them the determination to stay the course—or maybe they say, "Why fight if this is all I have to look forward to?" I must be a nightmare to some people. They could look at me and say, "My God! Is this what life will be like? Yes, she's surviving, but look at the hell she's gone through!"

⁂

I appreciate Carla for the best friend that she is, but also for all the things she's done for me over the years, like the Community Star nomination. When I turned forty-eight she surprised me with a huge memory book filled with cards, letters and photos from all sorts of people. One of my Baltimore oncologists flattered me with a note that said I was "the most courageous patient" he'd ever cared for. A grade school buddy reminded me of the May-pole dances we took part in at good old Easton School. There were tributes from relatives, co-workers, neighbors, and patients I'd come to know as friends over the years. It was an amazing gift and one that I cherish.

Judy and Linda are wonderful sisters too, but because Carla and I both live in Morgantown and work for the same company (she joined me there in 1993) we get to strengthen that bond on a daily basis. Sometimes at the end of the workday we'll hit the therapy pool just to relax. We hitch on the little flotation devices so we can goof around, dog-paddling like nincompoops while we chat about whatever comes to mind. It's a beautiful thing when sisterhood and true friendship intertwine!

Sweatin' to the Oldies

Before I was diagnosed with cancer I got plenty of physical exercise. For probably ten to fifteen years prior I had a solid walking routine. I did aerobics, jogged a bit, and even ran in the July Fourth race one year, although I was far from being an athlete. The other two women who were running the race with me became exhausted and had to quit, but I knew *I* had to finish. If I set my mind to something, I am filled with an almost ceaseless determination.

When I finally came through the shoot, more than six miles after the start of the race, there was no one at the finish line to greet me. Everyone had gone home. Dave said he was ready to send an ambulance along the path to look for me. It was a horrendous course, hilly and difficult. The weather was hot and antagonized the best of the runners. As I plodded across the line, an anonymous arm reached out and unceremoniously ripped the number tag off my chest.

I couldn't help the pathetic outcome! I'd even had to walk a little bit in order to complete the race. Despite this, I was thrilled to be listed only *next* to last. At his office the following day, someone was teasing Dave. They'd read the particulars on the race and noticed that Dave's wife brought up the tail end of the Fourth of July Race. "Hey, at least she finished," he said, defending my attempt, "At least she was *in* the race!" I was glad I'd taken part but never did it again. Instead, I stuck with my occasional two-mile run, nothing spectacular, just an enjoyable stretch. I was one of those people who's addicted to fun but not to exercise.

This hilly town is a great place for sledding when the snow's just right. Shortly after we moved into our current home I headed next door, a garbage can lid tucked under my arm, to ask my new neighbors if they'd like to hit the hills. They had a quizzical look on their faces. I know they probably wanted to say, "Aren't you just a tad too old for this?" but instead they were polite, "Well...um...guess we could see if the *kids* would like to go."

Even though Dave is "Mr. Golf," I have only gone with him once. That was enough for both of us. Never again. I kicked the ball.

I threw the ball. Anything to complete the tedious progression to the last hole. I was so bored and my arm hurt so much that at one point I'd asked Dave if we could please just leave. He wouldn't hear of it. "I paid for nine holes and we're golfing nine holes. Let's go!" In truth, he's probably relieved that I didn't become his golfing sidekick, tagging along with him on his get-away outings.

Neither am I cut out for the "Tour de Morgantown." Many times we've biked downtown from our house—just under four miles round trip. It was always easy going down. And it seemed to be just as easy for Dave on the return trip up the big hills. Not me. I'd be switching gears like crazy, trying mightily to balance the bike and sustain a bit of momentum.

One time I was so frustrated at my feeble attempt to negotiate the steep grade that I felt like crying. I yelled out to him, "I can't make it!" and flung the bike to the side of the street, ready to permanently abandon the contraption. He ignored me. Once I'd regained my composure I walked it up the hill. I was panting all the way, feeling like those unsuspecting flatland kids who enroll in WVU and double the size of their legs by midterm just walking to and from class.

Another Carrot in Formal Attire

Geoff was married in October of 1998. I was a little more involved in this wedding because his fiancée was a local girl whose parents we came to know over the nine years of our children's courtship. Geoff and Tricia were engaged in late December of 1997, on her birthday.

At the time of their marriage I was still taking Navelbine. I remember telling my doctor that I would need an extra week off so that I'd stand a better chance of feeling good at the wedding. There was no argument on his part, so I was "home free" as far as my protocol was concerned. The next question to consider: what to wear?

Every now and then a woman takes the liberty of indulging in a little "something special." For me, this was the dress I bought for Geoff's wedding. I'd seen it in a store here in town. It flirted with me from the hanger, winking that "Buy me! C'mon, buy me!" wink. I tried it on and was transformed from a middle-aged woman with cancer to a princess in a stunning gown. I didn't look like a cancer patient. I didn't feel like a cancer patient. And I didn't think I could afford the luxury of owning that sweet little thing—the kind of dress I'd only dreamed about wearing.

I'd gone shopping with Tricia's mother, Liz. We tried on dozens of dresses. We had a ball going from store to store and parading in front of the dressing mirrors. No matter what I put on, none gave me the same Cinderella feel. I kept returning to the dress shop and trying it on, just to tempt myself, I thought. One day I took my sister with me on my lunch hour. I slipped into the dressing room and came out modeling the dress I desperately wanted to take home, but knew I couldn't realistically afford.

"THAT'S the dress!" Carla assured me, in that "I'm your sister—listen to me!" tone. I put it back on the rack and left.

It was full-length with a long slit up the back. Sleeveless. V-neck. The shimmery little jacket that went with it had pearls embroidered on the trim in front. It was a luscious champagne color. Oh, to wear that dress. For the mother-of-the-groom to show up, chemo-free and looking like a million bucks! What might that feel like? I decided I had to find out.

After a talk with Dave I heard the musical words, "If you really want it, get it." He said, "This is a big day. You don't want to wear some other dress you don't really like, sorry that you left the other one hanging in the store."

That was all the inducement I needed. I went to the shop and made a down payment. The saleswoman seemed to have expected this outcome all along, "You wanted that dress the first day you came in here. It's perfect for you. I don't know why you bothered to try on anything else!" She was right. It was worth every indulgent penny.

Let's Have a Wedding

On the day Geoff and Tricia became husband and wife the sky was especially blue over our corner of the Mountain State. The generous sun warmed the October day to a lovely seventy-five degrees. It was gorgeous, the kind of weather that would make you happy even if you weren't already.

The wedding was in the late afternoon. When Dave and I arrived at the church we went downstairs to wait for the signal to come up for the ceremony. The photographer flitted around snapping pictures of us as we did our last minute primping and the clock ticked its last-minute ticking. With just minutes to go until we'd be escorted to our seats in the church, a loud thud startled us and drew our attention to the steps. Liz was lying at the bottom of the stairs in her beautiful mother-of-the-bride dress and newly ripped hose. Dave ran to her and tried to help her up, asking if she'd gotten hurt.

She couldn't stop laughing. "Are you okay? Are you sure you're okay?" Dave asked. Still she laughed, despite the fact that the slit in the front of her dress was now a little higher than it had been just moments before. Her knee was scraped. Her ankle was scraped. Her hose were destroyed. A pitiful sight, and yet, because Liz's laugh is so contagious, we all felt helpless to keep from joining in.

Our makeshift team of emergency personnel rushed her into the dressing room where Tricia was waiting. "Mom? What happened? Are you all right?" Her daughter asked worriedly.

"I caught my heel on the step and fell down," Liz answered, still smiling, as we packed one bag of ice on her knee and another on the injured ankle. Someone else fetched a pair of replacement nylons.

Just when we thought we'd had all the levity a near-tragedy can produce on such an occasion, one of God's little winged creatures crashed the party. A large bumblebee decided to investigate the hem of Tricia's long bridal veil during the ceremony. Afraid that the bee might crawl up on her head and cause an ugly scene, Dave made his move.

My husband, Navy Seal-like in his rescue attempt, and with the collective gaze of the wedding guests upon him, quietly edged near the bride without causing her to be distracted. In a quick move he snatched the bee from her "bonnet," creating just the slightest tug on the veil and making Tricia silently question what might possibly be happening behind her.

The rest of the wedding day was spared from any such catastrophic near misses. The reception was held at the Fairmont Field Club, where the splendor of the perfect autumn day could really be appreciated. As we approached the club, a gentleman stood on the hillside playing the bagpipes, the music greeting the guests with its timeless song, a tribute to the bride's Scottish grandmother. I wonder why it is that the sound of the pipes always seems to punctuate the air with a kind of simultaneous love and fear? Maybe it's the ageless struggle of the people who own that music, their struggle and proud survival. Or maybe it's my own.

It was music that touched us all later that day as well. After Tricia danced with her father, Geoff escorted me to the floor. Those guests who'd watched me dance with Greg at his wedding just two years earlier must have thought it a peculiar déjà vu. Me too, given that back in '96 I'd started a new chemo which wasn't working and was so sick even *Nancy Lofstead* had begun to doubt that her supply of resilience was, in fact, infinite.

When the song began, so did the tears that streamed down my son's face. For our dance together he'd chosen "You are the Sunshine of My Life." The emotion of the moment flowed across the room like ripples from a leaf dropped in water. As I looked at him and wiped his cheeks, I tried desperately to stay composed and prayed a mother's prayer of gratitude for the endurance that allowed me to experience that special day.

The guests who knew me well knew that I had reached another milestone. Those who did not would never have guessed I'd been battling ovarian cancer for nearly a decade and still undergoing chemo. For hours I danced and laughed, talked to people, and mingled about in my beautiful gown, all the while knowing that this particular "carrot" would soon become a part of the past. It was a wonderful day. What would I construe as the next carrot, the next immediate incentive to keep me looking forward, up instead of down? It's easy to hit a slump after a big event like your child's wedding. All of the excitement and planning slip quickly into scrapbooks and real life can start looking like a bare refrigerator to someone with an empty stomach.

Dial "M" for Mamaw

Our little family had successfully navigated another holiday season, remaining intact as I continued my chemo and stayed determined, and we happily added another Christmas stocking for our new daughter-in-law. 1999 rolled in with the usual bowl games and snowstorms. At work January was winding up to be a month for planning.

One day at the office my boss asked me to order some information from the American Physical Therapy Association for a seminar coming up in February. The A.P.T.A.'s phone order system is entirely automated. I dialed the number and punched in the appropriate codes for the materials we needed. Then a voice prompt said, "If you'd like to give your name with the order, key it in using the touchtone keypad on your phone." I thought I'd punched N-A-N-C-Y. That is, until about an hour later when a strange fax came through.

"Who is Mamaw?" a co-worker asked, especially puzzled.

I perked up, "What are you talking about?"

"Nancy, is there something you need to tell us?" she teased, "There's an A.P.T.A. fax here for someone named 'Mamaw'—hmm." We laughed.

I was embarrassed to give my boss the fax, who repeated the inquiry about Mamaw. "I'm afraid that's me," I said.

I assured the staff I wasn't hiding anything, and that, in fact, it would be impossible to hide my delight if I were to become a "Mamaw" or "Memaw" or "Nana"—any of the names befitting the rank of grandmother. I remembered thinking after Geoff's wedding, what will be the next carrot? Greg is married. Geoff is married. I'd seen them both graduate from college. I watched proudly as Greg earned his law degree and Geoff finished grad school. Wouldn't it be nice to have a grandchild? If becoming a grandparent could be my *next* carrot?

⸙

The night after the Mamaw fax I had just gone to bed when the phone rang. It was Greg, calling from their home in Charleston, South Carolina. His exact words to me were, "Mom, would you like to be called Grandma or Nana?" I jumped off the bed, and at the same time was screaming with surprise and crying. Dave immediately asked what was going on.

"Oh my gosh, Greg, is Jill pregnant?" I squealed.

Greg answered proudly, "Yes. We're having a baby!"

Their doctor had just confirmed what Jill had suspected at Christmastime but wasn't yet ready to announce. I told them about the funny fax and we all had a laugh. Their good news phone call meant I could sleep that night (and many more) knowing a darling "baby" carrot was dangling ahead of us. As for the fax, I've hung onto it as a reminder that we're sometimes given unlikely little previews of our future.

⸙

Little Ethan James could have become known to us as little "Floyd" if Mother Nature had gotten her way. Our grandson arrived on September 14th, not long before Hurricane Floyd ravaged the Carolinas. Jill's doctor had advised her to travel north to escape the storm. She gave Jill the file containing her medical records, along with the advice that any hospital anywhere could deliver her baby, blah, blah. Not very comforting news for a first-time mom, already two days overdue and living a long way from her Philadelphia family. The doctor's intended send-off was during an afternoon appointment on the 13th, about the same time the weather experts were beginning to predict a worrisome fate for Charleston.

The thought of taking part in a massive evacuation during a hurricane would freak out most people, but coupled with the anticipation of childbirth on the run, drive-up window-style, it was especially troublesome to Jill and Greg. They were up until midnight debating the pros and cons of leaving town versus staying put and "riding out the storm." Finally, they agreed to head out in the morning and went to bed to rest up for the trip.

But there would be no rest—Jill was soon having labor contractions. At 3:00 a.m. Greg drove down the empty streets of an abandoned Charleston to their hospital, one of the only spots that hadn't closed down. There his wife was assigned to the maternity ward's last available bed! Almost twelve hours after checking in, at the hands of the only obstetrician left in the hospital—a woman who was trying to deliver two other babies at the same time—Jill gave birth to sweet Ethan.

By then the city had undergone a mandatory evacuation. At 9:00 p.m. the hurricane "watch" had been upgraded to a "warning" for the entire South Carolina coast. No more cars were allowed to leave the city. The situation had become chaotic. The hospital lost power for a while and the phone lines were down. The jubilant "It's A Boy!" calls were postponed. Greg, Jill and Ethan were forced to spend their first few days as a family in a hospital room listening to the hurricane howl. Its winds brushed past the city peaking at more than eighty miles-per-hour (luckily, a far cry from Floyd's top speed of 155!).

At my suggestion they photographed Ethan in his bassinet lying next to a copy of the newspaper bearing headline news of the hurricane. Fortunately, Charleston was spared the brunt of the storm, experiencing mostly high winds and heavy rain. It wasn't long before Jill and Greg tired of all the jokes about their son not being named for the hurricane. "What? Not even his middle name is Floyd? (Perhaps if his birth had occurred one storm later, during one named Gunther or George, for instance...)

I absolutely could not wait to wrap my arms around this beautiful, tiny person who'd made me a grandmother. After finagling things just a bit and rearranging my chemo schedule (by now I had switched off of the Navelbine and resumed the Taxol infusions), we drove down in early October and met the little guy who had won our love long before we made his acquaintance.

It was an emotional experience, meeting for the first time this grandchild I'd thought I'd never live to see. I kept programming myself on the way down, "Nancy don't just grab the baby the instant you see him! Acknowledge Greg and Jill so they don't feel slighted." When we arrived Jill greeted us at the door with Ethan in her arms. I hugged her and said hello.

"Come on in and hold your grandson!" No other invitation could have made me happier.

I remember sitting down on the couch with him in my lap, just savoring this very special time. In the brief moment that followed, I recognized a feeling all too familiar to this mother of two. He'd peed on me.

"I see he's christened you," Jill chuckled.

We kept commenting on how much hair the little fellow had. During the months just prior, I'd lost most of mine in the process of going back on Taxol. Dave said, "Let's see which of the three of us has the most hair." Despite my balding dome, the snapshot clearly indicates I won that little contest.

Our initial visit with Ethan drove home the sense of creating another landmark in my life with cancer. Ten years earlier, when I was diagnosed, it seemed absolutely impossible that I'd survive long enough to see something I'd thought was so far out of reach—the birth of a grandchild. Even though I'd secretly hoped for the experience, it's not as if I could politely say to my sons, "Hurry up and get married, then have a baby because I might die soon!" Many times I'd wondered to myself, when are they going to have a child? I want so much to see a grandchild!

Unlike some people who don't welcome grandparenthood on the grounds it makes them seem old, I always wanted to be a grandma. I'd often heard it said that raising your kids is one thing, but being a grandparent is what's really special. Without the pressure of being a new parent it's easier to relax and enjoy their babyhood. You can hold them as long as you want and then hand them back, no looming responsibility to discipline or provide for them.

Ethan's arrival was one carrot, and an incredible one at that, but just having him in our lives and wanting to build a relationship with him means the carrot will be there for a long, long time. I think Dave and I realized the experience was not the same as it might have been for just any other couple. Our struggle prior to Ethan's birth really paved the way to absorb every ounce of joy he has to offer us. I see other couples with their grandchildren and question whether they appreciate those little ones as much as they would if mere survival itself were hanging in the balance.

For Dave, being a grandpa is extra special because he had a wonderful, close relationship with *his* grandfather. He's already planning the things they'll do together—fishing, golf. I know he can't wait to place a putter in the baby's hands and start giving him some tips. Dave looks forward to the talks they'll have—buddies from the get-go.

Picking Flowers

Throughout my illness I've often drawn support from my mother. She reassured me many times during these difficult years that prayer held the power to work miracles. Whenever I returned to her side, familiar to me since childhood, she offered her own brand of comfort. I can still hear her consoling words, "We'll pray about it." She kept me focused on the greater scheme of life, and the power that was greater than the combined strength of all of us flawed mortals. Not one to coddle, she taught by example and raised us to be independent.

Still, I felt I could tell her anything. I confided in her about matters that I knew would burden almost anyone else, "Mom, I'm soooo sick of this!" I'd openly complain about whatever happened to be causing my suffering on that given day, "I'm tired Mom. I can't stand this anymore!" She never stopped being my mother. One fall day I was ill and left work to go home and rest. Once there I plugged in the humidifier, trying to get more moisture in the house to ease my symptoms. I called her, "Mom, I need you."

"What do you need Nancy?" she asked, willing to accommodate almost any request.

"I'm home in bed. The humidifier's running but I need another one. I'm still having trouble breathing. I've got to get more moisture in the air."

"Your dad and I will be right over." And they were. She sat at the bottom of my bed for two or three hours and we watched TV as I rested. Like clockwork, at the prescribed hour, she announced, "Time to change the channel now. *Jeopardy!* is on. You know I never miss *Jeopardy!*."

My parents met before World War II when they were both involved in exhibition roller-skating. Terrific skaters, they performed as a skating duo to the delight of crowded audiences. My dad skated here ages ago in an exhibition at the historic Hotel Morgan.

Eventually they decided the roller rink wasn't all they had in common. Before he headed off to fight he slipped an engagement ring on her finger, holding a graceful young hand that bore no sign of the crippling arthritis that would later turn it into a tangle of pain.

On the night she died, Dad had heard Mom fall to the floor and went to help her. This was not an uncommon chain of events. She was often so stiff and in so much pain that it was difficult for her to walk and keep her balance. Many times he had rescued her from these falls, methodically reaching under her upper arms and pulling her to a seated position on the floor. Then she'd brace herself against his body as she slowly rose to her feet and kept leaning on him as he helped her back into bed.

He still questions how he was able to do it. How, on that particular night, his nearly eighty-year-old frame summoned the strength of a champion skater, as he LIFTED his beloved Jean from the floor onto her bed. Our family still talks about the mystery of that act, knowing full well that the power of deep love gives our bodies the strength to accomplish almost anything our hearts can imagine.

As for myself, I will always consider that Mom knew she would soon leave us. I was eager to have her meet Ethan, but that moment would never arrive. In a phone call on the Tuesday night before Thanksgiving I'd told her about a young cancer cousin who'd just lost her battle, survived by a husband and darling three-year-old daughter. Mom remembered the family from our previous discussions. She'd lived through each of the stories of my cancer cousins with me. I knew she wasn't going to cry on the phone when I needed someone to be strong and listen to me grieve over the loss. I always felt free to share these friendships with her. "Mom, I met another lady today with ovarian cancer…Mom, I just found out another woman I've been supporting is going in for more surgery…Another friend has died, Mom."

In response to the story of the young mother, she offered an unusual flicker of philosophy. Mom extended her understanding with a simple statement, "Nancy, God plants those flowers and God chooses when to pick them."

On the way home from work the next night I picked up my cell phone and gave her a call. I was so excited to be hosting our family's celebration. I told her about the dinner I was planning. She mentioned that they'd be bringing two pies, "Apple and pumpkin. We'll try to be there about noon."

Just hours later, before the autumn dawn could cast its light on another Thanksgiving, God entered His garden again, this time choosing one very dear bloom.

An Element of Surprise

Reaching my 50th birthday in 2000 was a true milestone. Having been diagnosed at thirty-nine, then puking my way through my 40th, I was as shocked as anyone that I was around to cross off those last few weeks that lead me to the half-century mark. I think this birthday can be especially difficult for women. They think about fifty and see wrinkles, see the face of a clock that ticks louder than ever before, are forced to admit they are most certainly on the downhill slope of anything resembling youth, at least according to the numbers.

Not me. I didn't care about wrinkles. I didn't care if I looked old. I wanted very much to hit fifty. I want very much to grow old. Each year is a medal of honor when you're duking it out with cancer.

Dave's 50th was two days before mine, on a Saturday. That morning he said he felt like hitting some golf balls. It was a cold, dreary February day, the kind that lets that cozy "weekend feeling" resonate with a special sweetness. I told him to go have fun. He and his buddy headed to an indoor driving range to kill a couple of hours. The morning outing would be part of his birthday celebration that would continue when we went out to dinner that night.

Out of the blue my friend Jan called and said she wanted to take me to lunch. I was game: nothing else was shakin' on my Saturday afternoon agenda. She explained that lunch was to celebrate my birthday and that our other friend, Marsha, would join us. Cool. A meal out with the girls, I thought. She asked where I'd like to eat, suggesting Back Bay, a local seafood place. Because Dave and I had just eaten there recently, I countered with a place out at the mall called Garfield's. She made some excuse and again suggested eating at Back Bay. "Fine, if you really want to, I don't care," I said.

I dressed and waited for her. When Jan arrived to pick me up something seemed a bit odd. Even though she'd been to my home many times, she was taking a keen interest in our antiques. We've always had antiques, it seems. When we were first married and trying to make ends meet, the only pieces of furniture we could afford were purchased from Dave's grandparents, "Pop" and Grandma Stout, who sold antiques. We'd occasionally pick out a piece or two and then whittle a few dollars off of our running tab as funds allowed—or "splurge" after an income tax refund or bonus check.

"You know, that's a really nice little piece of furniture," Jan commented, pointing at something I'd had for years, "When did you get that?"

"Oh I've had that a while. C'mon, let's get going. Marsha's going to be waiting for us," I answered impatiently.

Jan continued, "You know, I really don't remember you having that. Now when exactly did you get it?"

When we were finally seat-belted in the car and heading out, I found myself wondering why she was driving so slowly and pointing out all of the real estate signs and points of interest along the route.

Eventually we made it across town to the seafood restaurant. I hadn't remembered that they're not open for lunch on the weekends, just for dinner, and not until around four or five. She pulled the car near the front door and told me to hop out. "No, that's okay. Go park and I'll walk in with you," I offered.

"No, go ahead and get out here," she insisted.

"Really, it's okay, I don't mind walking," I told her. "Hey, look over there," I pointed across the parking lot, "Somebody must be having a party, there's a guy carrying a gift."

Then she got pushy. "Get out of the car Nancy. It's your birthday and I want to let you out at the front door." Geez! What's the big deal? I wondered, suspecting at last that something bizarre might be going on.

When I got through the front door I spotted my niece's boyfriend with a video camera. "Hi Michael. What the heck are you doing here?" I asked. He didn't answer. "Miiiike…what - are - you - doing?" I repeated as I looked around the room, adding, "Something's not right here!" At that point I wanted to turn and run out the door. I'm not one for surprises. I like to be in control and know what's coming and I hadn't keyed in on this one.

"SURPRISE!!!" a multitude of familiar voices yelled from the balcony. I immediately started to cry. I walked up the steps and was embraced by my sister Judy, who'd made the long trip in from Cleveland. Linda drove all the way over from Dayton. My dad was there. Carla. I couldn't stop hugging people. There were so many friends and relatives there to cheer me across the threshold of my fifty years. I was really moved. I got a closer look at the man from the parking lot who'd carried the present, *my* present, and recognized him as one of our friends.

Jan finally came into view. She explained that she'd gotten a call from Dave to stall me if possible, that folks were running late and he needed more time. A dedicated accomplice indeed!

There were childhood friends there that I'd met more than forty years ago. It was so touching to see those lifelong pals. It sounds trite to say, "Where does the time go?" But I'm convinced it was just yesterday that we'd mischievously entertained ourselves, victimizing the Easton School restrooms with sloppy wads of wet tissue that stuck perfectly like globs of plaster to the high ceiling.

One of the guests was a cancer patient I'd hooked up with. She'd driven hours from the southern part of the state to help me celebrate. There were people from work. People from Harner Chapel. People from everywhere, even one of my chemo nurses from the Cancer Center.

With help from my sister Carla, Dave had planned out the whole afternoon. I don't know how they did it. They'd ordered a decorated cake and trays of hors d'oeuvres. We had a great time. Dad was nearly as excited as I was. He knew so many of the people there. I'd walk up to him with one of the old school chums, "Dad, do you remember who this is?" And most of the time he got the name right. It was like a reunion of sorts. I couldn't believe Dave and Carla had gotten around to calling ALL these people!

Many of the guests made entries in a little birthday journal that was passed around at the party that afternoon. I treasure it as a keepsake of that most special day. I still like to go back and read the greetings and recall the happiness and gratitude I felt.

As my chemo nurse was saying good-bye, she waved cheerfully, "See ya Friday!"

"Oh, by the way, I'll need to call you about that. I need to reschedule my chemo this week." I said. She looked puzzled. I added, "I'm going roller-skating on Saturday and I want to make sure I feel good."

She leaned over and whispered to me, "Well Nancy, you just let us know when we can schedule your chemo around the roller-skating." I promised I would!

When we left the restaurant, my sisters and I headed to Dad's place. There, his four girls sat around the kitchen and talked and laughed for hours. We ordered pizza for dinner. Our dad doesn't hear well, and for the most part didn't know what we were discussing. He was happy just to watch our animated conversation fill his warm home, as *he* filled with the sense of contentment that comes from knowing certain bonds endure a lifetime.

As I fell to sleep that cold night, feeling like a kid who's had more candy and fun than she could stand, I couldn't help but consider the sheer excitement of the celebration. Focused on me, of all people, and *my* big "five-O" and my nearly eleven years of cancer survival. And all this on the same day of my selfless husband's 50th birthday! A night for sweet dreams if ever there was one.

Here a Cancer, There a Cancer, Everywhere a Cancer

All those childhood days spent playing with my brother D.L. and my sisters for long hours in the hot sun have taken their revenge on this adult body. Splashing around in the pond out at Chestnut Ridge Park until I was a roasty-toasty shade of pink has forced me to deal with basal cell carcinoma on top of everything else. Back in those days we just poured on the Coppertone and let the all-day picnic begin! I never thought about sunscreen or the risks involved with my many burn-blister-peel sequences.

In fact, I have many fond memories of those days…Mom and our neighbor lady played Scrabble and kept an eye on us from under the big oak tree, not far from the pond's sandy shore. In between our water adventures we'd head to the blankets the two mothers had spread out on the ground for us. We'd gobble down homemade sandwiches from the coolers and sip cold drinks from shiny aluminum tumblers.

Mom was an excellent swimmer. As a kid she'd almost *lived* in the pool near her family's home in Mannington and even worked there as a lifeguard. She loved the water and looked fantastic in a bathing suit, even years after giving birth to her son and four daughters. I didn't inherit my mother's command of the water. It took three sets of swimming lessons before I mastered the basics. Her home movie of my debut on the diving board is a funny reminder of my girlish trepidation.

There I am in the flickering frame, heading one skinny foot in front of the other down the diving board (which might just as well have been a gangplank over the high seas). Then I disappear from the frame. Mom has now refocused the movie camera on the surface of the pool, thinking I've somehow already made my dive. Still no Nancy. Back to the diving board, filming from tip to ladder…there her nervous daughter fills the frame again, obviously rethinking the wisdom of such a plunge!

I didn't manage to inherit Mom's skin either. After all her years in the sun there were harmless pigmentation marks dotting her arms and legs, but none of the basal cell that's speckled my medical records.

By now I've had so many little spots cut off here and there that it's really no big deal when another one pops up. The skin cancer is my "ace in the hole." Say I'm whining to a co-worker about how I can't help out with something because I have cancer, blah, blah, blah. If I'm not getting the desired effect, I throw in the tidbit about the blood clot in my jugular vein. Still a big "So What!?" Then I trot out the basal cell and figure they've gotta cut me some slack.

One day I was in getting my chemo and thought I might as well kill two birds with a single stone. After everything was safely underway I stood up and said to the dismayed nurses, "Okay girls, I'll see ya later. Time to go visit the dermatologist." I looped the I.V. tubing up around the pole and wheeled my skinny metal companion down the hall.

"What have we got here?" the doctor asked.

"I'm getting my chemo," I answered, hoping he'd go along with my plan. I'd even dressed for the occasion, wearing sweat pants with shorts underneath to make it easier for him to examine my legs. I had six spots for him to check. When he determined that five of them would have to come off I ordered him to commence slicing.

"No. I'm not going to do that to you anymore," he said, explaining that he'd rather freeze them off.

"C'mon. Just numb the little devils and grab your scalpel. I've got the insurance authorization for a 'Visit With Biopsy.' Get to it!"

"No. I just can't cut on you anymore. I've done it too many times," he refused. He was right. I have scars on my upper thigh, on my back, my rib cage, my chest, the back of my hand, my forearm, and my shoulder. If I tried, I could probably connect the dots and come up with a fairly intricate constellation.

On the way home that day I remarked to Dave that I probably wouldn't get much mileage out of this latest episode, "These wimpy little freezer burns aren't going to garner nearly as much sympathy as the gross-looking surgical scars!" He agreed. They weren't even in places where I could easily show them off.

A couple summers ago I had two exceptionally large basal cells removed from my leg. My low white count interferes with my ability to heal quickly and so, for a long while, those two spots were the nastiest looking sores you've ever seen. As if following a script, people would see the spots and say, "Oh my gosh! What on earth happened to your leg?"

I'd whip out my handy tale about a big fat man who sat on the bleacher in front of us at a ball game. I'd tell how he leaned back and accidentally extinguished his cigar on my leg! When that wore out, I referred to the locusts swarming noisily all over town that summer. "A giant locust attacked me!" I fibbed. "Before I even knew what was happening the little sucker bored right down into my leg!"

When I ran out of creative explanations I'd confess that the problem was really basal cell carcinoma, but no one seemed to find that nearly as interesting. No one except my primary care physician, who was shocked by the sight of the ugly scars and didn't fall for *either* cigars or locusts.

Maybe the inclination toward tall-tales is genetic. When Geoff was just a pre-schooler, one of his babysitters, a rather stern older woman, implied that we'd been neglectful parents for not preventing the dog attack that scarred his little tummy. Well, that's what he told *her*, anyway, choosing not to reveal that the scar was from an abdominal surgery he'd had as an infant. Chip off the old block, eh?

The removal of my very first basal cell growth was no laughing matter. It was on my eyelid! It happened back in 1993. I recall grilling the doctor just before she helped me up off the operating table to go look in the mirror.

"Now, there won't be a big scar, will there?"

"No, no, no," she answered.

"It's not going to bruise a lot, is it?"

"It'll be okay," she said calmly.

"Will people be able to see it?"

"Don't worry," she said, taking me by the arm.

When I met the image in the mirror I freaked out. "Oh my God! Look at that!"

"Everything will be fine," she reassured me, "It will heal soon."

She'd had to make a V-shaped incision downward from the lower lid to release a tiny muscle and remove the basal cell. It was not a pretty sight. I told inquiring minds I'd simply had a little eye tuck for cosmetic reasons, and that if it turned out well I might have the other eye done. When John and Sabra's son asked what was wrong with my eye, I saw the chance to spin a good one.

"Well, Tim, you know how the price of lettuce has been so high lately?"

"Yeah."

"Well, I just happened to be out at the Giant Eagle the other day when it was announced over the store intercom that lettuce was being marked down to just fifty-nine cents a head. No limit!"

"Yeah?"

"Tim, I'm telling you it became a battle scene!" His eyes widened in anticipation of my next line, "This lady grabbed a head of lettuce right out of my hand and then some other ladies started throwing lettuce. It was unbelievable! One of them hit me right in the eye!"

"No way!" he exclaimed. "At the Giant Eagle store?"

I really had him going until Sabra made me 'fess up to the surgery, which in itself was stranger than fiction.

At the time I was still going through the phase where I'd do anything to avoid getting an I.V. When my doctor asked ahead of time if I'd need anything to relax on the day of the eye surgery, I declined, knowing the "relaxant" would have to be fed through a needle inserted in my arm.

"Nope. I'll just come on downstairs from the clinic, climb up on the table and you can cut this off," I proclaimed confidently, picturing myself bravely boarding our fourth floor elevator at the clinic and zipping into our office.

"Well, let me at least give you some Valium," she offered.

"Okay," I agreed, "But I probably won't need it."

She instructed me to take one pill at 9:00 that morning and another one at 9:30. I took the first one right on schedule but didn't feel anything happen. A half hour later I swallowed the second one and almost immediately started inviting co-workers to come downstairs with me and watch the surgery, "C'mon guys, it'll be fun!"

I proceeded down at the proper time, by myself, happy as a lark. The nurse instructed me to undress and slip into a hospital gown. I flatly refused. "No thanks. There will be no gown for me. I'm going to climb up on the table in my own clothes and get this over with quickly." After a bit more negotiation I found myself dressed in the stylish gown and firmly declining an I.V. sedative.

"That's not necessary," I told her. "I want to be awake for this."

Once I was finally on the table she started to numb the area around my eye with Novocain or Xylocaine or something. I couldn't feel anything. Then they started to drape me for the surgery. I thought it was a funny scene, my whole body covered except for this big, disembodied eyeball staring out at them and around the room.

I was strapped down to the table and someone was holding my hand. In a minute I FELT the cut into my skin when the doctor started to make the incision. I didn't want to let her know I felt it so I pretended nothing was happening—this can't be any worse than getting an I.V., right? I'll tough it out.

As she proceeded I tried desperately to conceal the pain but my feet rose in unison as high as the restraints would allow. I started humming. Nothing in particular, just any song I could think of to help keep my mind occupied.

The doctor paused, "Nancy, do you *feel* this?"

"Oh no. No, go right ahead," I lied.

In a short while, when my feet couldn't raise any higher and I'd hummed every song ever written, I broke down and told her I was in pain. They numbed the area a bit more and she continued, digging deeper than she'd originally planned, diligently trying to snatch every particle of the basal cell in the process. That's when she explained she'd have to cut the little muscle. It would allow the eyelid to drop down so that she could get it all. I already knew this was coming, because there had been a knock at the door and a voice telling her "the margins are not clean."

"I heard that!" I'd said.

"I know you did. Sorry, but I have to cut deeper," she apologized.

With this even my knees were starting to come up off the table and, not wanting to scream, the humming got louder.

"Could you please stop humming, Nancy?" she asked firmly. Guess I was throwing off her concentration.

Eventually the surgery was over. I don't know which of us was happier. I'd thought I was tough, having gone through all the previous surgeries and procedures. But I was naïve, so determined that I could get by without the I.V. anesthesia, and certainly without the embarrassment of the excessive gagging and vomiting. Luckily for me, she was a compassionate doctor who understood the emotional side of such physical ramifications. Later this gifted woman would face her own cancer enemy, succumbing less than four months after diagnosis.

A Best Friend

Winston has been a great companion to Dave and me during the years of my struggle with cancer. Unfortunately in my case, as most pet owners will tell you, animals know when something's up. If I'm sick, Winston sleeps on the floor on my side of the bed, otherwise he's on the opposite side near the "master" of the house. Boxers are known for being both loyal and loving pets and he certainly matches that description.

Winston makes us laugh. At times he's like a big clumsy kid who will never grow up. The colorful bandanas we tie around his neck give him the look of a Jimmy Buffet fan club member. Winston has a habit of twitching and snoring in his sleep. In fact, he can sound rather human-like. At times I've been known to give Dave a little nudge with my elbow to get him to quit snoring, only to later discover it's a four-legged nocturnal disturbance.

Winston doesn't seem to like it when Geoff and Tricia bring their two Labs, McKenzie and Barclay, to visit. All three dogs are fun pets, but Winston wants this turf to himself—no competition! The Labs stay out at Tricia's parents in the country where they have plenty of room to run around the yard. Tricia has a plaque that says "dogs are just children with fur." It's true the mutts certainly work their way into your heart...and your vehicle. They live in Michigan where Geoff's the tournament director for the Michigan Section of PGA of America. In order to make the long trips back to Morgantown with the dogs, they had to buy a cargo carrier for their Jeep. There's no way the luggage would fit in back with the two rambunctious Labs.

Winston gets very upset when I have to be hospitalized. He knows when Dave comes home alone that it must mean trouble for me. Winston will pace nervously around the house and garage looking for me, denying the obvious fact that I won't be spending the night as usual, home with the two of them. I'll never forget how agitated he was the time Jan came over to rescue me from the shaking attack that came over me in the tub. He put Jan under close scrutiny to make sure I wasn't being harmed. It's sad that not even our dog has been spared from the stress of my disease.

Each time I'm released from the hospital it seems Winston is just as happy and relieved as the rest of us. When he sees me making my way up the sidewalk he gets excited and heads for the front door to welcome me. His big brown eyes can say so much. There is no doubt in my mind when it comes to the debate over pets and their sensitivity to emotions. How lucky I am to have even the love and support of our pup in this difficult journey!

CHAPTER 6

Something in the Air

2001

Flying the Friendlier Skies

Always eager to spend time with my grandson Ethan, I planned a trip to South Carolina for Dad and me this past spring. The trip was a real "pick-me-up" for my father *and* me. While Dad was happy to be seeing both baby and parents, he was also psyched up for the flight itself. Who could blame him? It would be his first since his days as a waist gunner in World War II!

He told me many times about the sensation of lying flat in the "waist" of the bomber, waiting for the right moment to stand up and take his position with the gun pointed out the open window. This inaugural trip on a passenger plane was fascinating for him. I teased him as we boarded, "Now Dad, don't be lying down in the aisles. This isn't a B-17. There are lots of comfy seats on *this* plane."

He was like a little kid who simply couldn't take it all in. And there's a lot of kid left in him! A while back we took a family roller skating trip to Point Marion, Pennsylvania—just a few miles from here—where we used to skate as kids. My eighty-one-year-old dad was speeding around the rink with more ease than skaters half his age, his signature bolo tie flying as he passed us.

During our flight Dad was intrigued with everything from the tiny windows and their pull-down plastic covers to the nifty barf bags and tray tables. It was a joy to watch him take in this new experience. He quizzed the flight attendant who seemed pleased with herself for remembering all the right answers.

"What make is this airplane?"

"Where was it manufactured?"

"How fast are we going?"

"How high are we?"

After hearing that it was his first venture into the air since the War, she graciously invited him up into the cockpit when we landed. He chatted with the pilots. "Things look a little different than I remember them!" he joked, as they pointed out the computerized instruments.

Dad loves to travel, and is always recalling what a great time he and Mom had taking off for the Southwest on extended vacations, the two of them stopping to sightsee and pick up turquoise pieces that they came across here and there. We all miss her, but I'm sure the loss of her companionship is especially tough on Dad. He often reflects on their vacations, "We had some great trips, that's for sure! We made the most of our time together—you can't take that away from us!"

We had a nice visit with Greg and Jill and little Ethan. As always, the time passes way too fast on excursions like these. I treasure every minute I can spend with my grandson and hope that he'll have some memory of these times when he's a grown-up. I'd always pictured myself as a funny old grandmother, playing with the kids and doing goofy things to make them laugh, the way I entertained my nieces and nephews, flipping pancakes high into the air and catching them on the spatula, playing jokes and so on. Never did I imagine myself in a rocking chair, much less a wheelchair!

I was glad to be doing a bit of traveling this spring. Last year at this same time I was making the switch from Taxol to a new chemo, Gemzar. My muscles and joints had begun to ache after a year and a half of the Taxol infusions and more important, the tumor marker was climbing as well.

On the way home to Morgantown we hit a hearty batch of turbulence. We were sitting in the first row of seats. My feet were planted firmly against the bulkhead. I worried that Dad might be nervous. I glanced at him and saw that he'd closed his eyes.

"Sure is shakin' the old toolbox," he grinned without blinking.

We'll be home before long, I thought. I closed my eyes too, letting my mind wander off to the safe and peaceful place where all good fathers want their children to be.

Fun and Games with Dr. Oncologist

I'll have to say that throughout this cancer ordeal my relationship with most of my doctors has been out of the ordinary. I'd venture to guess most patients haven't gone shopping for their doctor's spouse, or for that matter, attended a major league baseball game right after a check-up. See what I mean?

Back in the early 1990s, when I was still taking the Tamoxifen, I was planning a visit to Baltimore for a routine follow-up. During a previous visit my doctor had suggested that Dave and I catch an Orioles game with him next time around. Being the good sports buffs that we are, we took him up on the offer and decided to schedule my appointment after checking the home game schedule. We figured the match-up against the Cleveland Indians ought to be a good one and called to make my appointment. Even though the game was on a Thursday and his clinic days fell on Wednesday, my doctor waved us in, assuring us he could set us up for both.

He met us at the clinic wearing his lab coat and looking professional as always. Things went well at the exam. Then he instructed us to go grab a bite and meet him at the Utah Street entrance to Camden Yards. His wife was out of town, so in her place he was bringing along a guy who was completing a medical illustrator internship. We changed clothes at his office then headed out to Fuddrucker's for our meal. It was a hot August day. The Tamoxifen made me sweat. We waited at the entrance gate, roasting in the sun, until we finally spotted him, or someone who looked like him.

The man who approached bore only a slight resemblance to the doctor we'd just talked to at the clinic. He was wearing plaid shorts. He was wearing white knee socks that had red stripes at midcalf. His shirt was striped. His tennis shoes had seen their better days. He was carrying a briefcase crammed with papers. And to top it all off, on his head he wore a ball cap with the logo "OB-GYN Construction Co." The illustrator, on the other hand was dressed fairly well. He looked nothing like his ballpark benefactor.

"Ya ready to go?" my doctor shouted.

"You bet," we chimed in.

He handed over the four tickets at the gate and bulldozed his way up the long ascent toward the box seats that would house our tired fannies once we got there.

"Hey, slow down. I have cancer, you know. I can't keep up with you guys in this heat," I complained.

"Aw c'mon," he said, jeering. "You can make it!"

"*You're* the one who gave me the Tamoxifen," I said accusingly. "It's the reason I can't handle this heat! I'm burning up."

He literally tore through that stadium to our section. Once we all rendezvoused there, Dave offered to pay him for the great seats, but the doctor wouldn't hear of it. He agreed only to the treat of a beer and hotdog. Between innings he pulled wads of paper from his briefcase and scribbled hasty notes on the pages, talking to us as he did so.

The rest of us looked up enough to see that the sky was clouding over and a rainstorm was about to hit. We stood in the concourse during the eventual downpour, waiting for the "rain delay" status to be lifted from the game. Finally, the whole game was called off. The doctor apologized, but we knew there was nothing anyone could do. We thanked him for his generosity and headed to the car, parked in the convenient, little known hideaway he'd directed us to. On the way, Dave and I laughed at the whole crazy day. We splashed each other as we stomped through the rain-filled mud puddles en route to the car.

⚮

Although it's far from a life and death issue, I am secretly grateful the man *I* married does not mix his stripes and plaids. The doctor may have realized his gift was in medicine and not necessarily in clothes shopping because he once asked me to buy a blazer for his wife. At first I couldn't believe I'd heard him correctly.

"You know that jacket of yours my wife likes?" he asked.

"Yes," I said.

"I want her to have one for a birthday present."

"But I don't think I could find it out here," I explained. "I bought it at a shop called The Finery back in Morgantown."

"No problem," he said. "Here's my credit card. Would you pick one up and mail it to her?"

⚮

Later on, even his office secretary got in on the baseball deal. Dave and I made it over to see a couple games with Barb and her husband. We got a hold of some Oriole tickets and stayed at a nice hotel in the Inner Harbor. It was fun walking down to the games and taking part in America's favorite pastime.

One of the games was in 1996, about the time my doctors and I suspected the cancer had spread to my bones. Oncology, Orioles, why not combine the two? Might as well see a game while we're in town. Maybe it would lift our spirits, we rationalized. Dave booked a beautiful harbor hotel for the night.

I remember how much fun the four of us had the time it was "hat night" at the stadium. The Orioles played the White Sox. One of the brewing companies was giving out free "Gilligan"-type hats at the gate. We all agreed to wear one so we could take part in the theme. Sporting our dopey hats, we just kicked back in the warm sun, a few rows from the first-base line, the guys each drinking a cold beer, and Barb and I enjoying our ice cream. Cancer doesn't have to be *all* bad, I thought, checking out the scoreboard, fiddling with my hat and ignoring the medical news of the day.

Driving Miss Nancy

In June of 2000 our clinic moved from its rented hospital floor into a brand new facility, tripling its size from about 12,000 to 36,000 square feet and adding a large therapy pool and lap lanes. From the humble beginnings of a one-therapist office, the clinic, now called "HealthWorks," has around sixteen full-time physical therapists and a full staff of auxiliary personnel, not to mention branch clinics in three other cities. Someone told me the other day that our payroll now numbers 115—a far cry from the staff of three in 1980!

My co-worker Mike and I were placed in charge of coordinating the transition to the new location. I knew that when moving day came I'd be on my feet a lot but didn't feel quite strong enough to walk around the building all day long. I'd even changed my chemo schedule to make sure I'd feel my best for the move.

My dad held the key to the solution. He suggested I borrow the electric cart he'd purchased for my mom. Her twenty-five years of rheumatoid arthritis had made it especially difficult for her to get around. The cart had allowed her the freedom to take part in camping trips or to go shopping. Dad simply loaded the little machine in and out of the back of their van as needed. He was happy to bring it "out of mothballs" and hand me the keys. With one small stipulation, that is.

Dad had spent his working life behind the counter of the Morgantown Post Office, weighing packages to the nearest ounce, counting out change to the penny, and strictly adhering to both the letter and spirit of the laws governing the mighty U.S. Postal Service. To say he places a certain value and priority on doing things right, by the book, and with respect for the relevant rules is a bit of an understatement.

So when I talked about borrowing "the wheels" he was very quick to say, "Oh that's fine. If it will help you, no problem. However, you'll need to come over so I can show you how to operate it." I agreed, thinking, there's surely not too much to operating a little electric cart, right? You just push the little handle to go, let off the little handle to stop. I went out to his place one evening and watched as he carefully wheeled it out of the garage with a reverence one might show toward a tiny ancient replica of the Trojan Horse.

�֍

In an instant I was having flashbacks to my early driving lessons. Dad had purchased a Volkswagen bus with a stick shift for me to drive to high school. He methodically taught me to master its tricky manual transmission. Eventually I did okay, despite the vicarious anxiety that had built up in me from earlier watching my older sister Linda at the wheel of the family car.

I can still envision my siblings and me packed nervously into the backseat on the way to Grandma's. En route, Linda at the wheel of the five-speed, it seems we always managed to hit the crest of the big hill at a most inopportune moment. With her tentative foot stammering between clutch and accelerator, we'd jabber a collective silent prayer, "Pleaseletthelightstaygreen. Pleaseletthelightstaygreen. PLEASEletthelightstaygreen!"

Unable to contain her tension, Mom had demanded of her mate, "Honestly Rich, why do you make her take this route?"

If we happened to witness the green/GO! skip from amber/CAUTION!! to red/STOP!!!, a chorus of sighs filled the car as Linda downshifted and hit the brakes. Determined to not let her family roll backward down the hill and into sure demise, Linda would trounce the gas pedal with all her weight as we counted down to blast-off, the engine's loud vibration buzzing through the car with the grind of a low-flying blender. In the end, she had mastered the manual transmission, but without the conviction that our brother D.L. had when he later took up auto racing. No question, Dad's a man with motives.

❧

On the day of my cart lesson he began, "Now first, Nancy, I want you to see how we connect and disconnect everything." He'd had it plugged in to charge the battery, so he showed me in detail how to unplug it, how to tuck in the cord, put the cover back over the battery, and so forth. I went through all the detailed steps, careful not to hit the wrong switch and launch a nuclear arsenal or commit some other fateful blunder. Then my father instructed me to 1) drive it up the driveway, 2) turn it around, and 3) come back to the garage. I followed his instructions, making sure I didn't put it in high speed. "Leave it in five or six, Nancy," he called after me. I complied.

Then, in the manner of a trainer at a kennel show, he instructed me to drive through the yard, over the sidewalk, and down to the garage. I did everything in sequence and followed every one of his instructions, feeling all the while like a little fifty-year-old child. Relieved that my driving lesson was finally over, I zipped back into the garage, where, just for a second, I lost track of the fact that I was supposed to *let off* the handle to stop it. But it only takes a second...

Instinctively, I put my feet out on both sides, dragging them to try to slow the strong-willed cart. I ran into a couple jugs of water before I managed to come to a complete halt. "You're going to hurt someone," he warned. There was only one way to deal with the matter.

I had to start the lesson all over again—from scratch. *From scratch!* Humbled, I began by plugging the charger cord back into the wall and then unplugging it, listening to his instruction as I did so. I had to go through the entire lesson again—just because I put my feet out instead of letting off the break handle. I must have been out there an hour. When we finished he said, "Now are you *sure* you know how to do it?" I promised him I could handle it, mustering the earnestness of a refugee begging for citizenship.

Moving day came. The parking lot of the new facility served as the drop-off point for the goods in question. Dad delivered the cart and unloaded it, wanting to know if I needed to go over the features again. I politely declined, "No I think I can do it, Dad." Soon I was on my own. I didn't dare let anyone get on the cart. It terrified me to think that someone might abuse it or run over someone, causing a serious injury or broken leg. I didn't recall feeling this nervous the first time I'd headed out to the movies driving the family car.

Shaken by his doubt in my competence, I repeated a short mantra as I started out, "I feel very comfortable. I'm going to be fine." I drove it all day. I'd planned ahead. There was a little wire basket in front, which I loaded with miniature candy bars. As I drove around the clinic, checking on stations here and there, seeing how the movers were doing, how people were settling into their areas, like a portable welcome wagon unit, I offered my good wishes along with candy from the basket.

At the end of the day I had to secure it in an area that was locked. I found a small office on the main floor and secreted the machine into a sort of overnight safe deposit box. "Plug it in so it can charge," I commanded myself, "Don't forget to plug it in!" Then, making sure I had the keys and that it was in the "off" position, I gave myself permission to leave the premises. The next morning I went immediately to the office to confirm that it was still secure.

I returned the equipment intact. Dad must have been proud of me. And I was grateful to him. It was the biggest help to have the cart! I went all day long and wasn't tired. I don't know that I would ask to use it again, though…I might have to go through a recertification in order to get the keys!

A Summer Storm

It happened without any warning, my latest tussle with chemo and its awful side effects. I'd been hoping to have a good summer following a spring that went fairly well—along with the trip to visit Ethan, the season had even included a neat Caribbean cruise for Dave and me in March. We went with Pat and Liz (Geoff's in-laws) and had a great time out on the water. But one never knows what's around the next bend in these mountain roads, or what's ahead when the time comes to switch to another chemo.

Last fall, when my tumor marker had again shown a significant increase, my doctor substituted my prescription for Gemzar with one for Topotecan, which I hadn't taken since 1997. With this go-round I would get a once a week Topotecan infusion rather than the four-day-long, once-a-month protocol of '97. Things were going okay until it became clear the Topotecan was not helping me. Now June of 2001 had arrived, along with the need for yet another switch in my chemo.

I'd taken some Valium to relax before I went in for the infusion of the new drug because I was a bit nervous about trying this chemo for the first time. Its name alone—Carboplatin—brought apprehension into my gut. It sounded too much like the old warhorse chemo (Cisplatin) that had made me desperately ill years earlier. The Valium was a small dose, just a couple milligrams, but it really put me in a stupor. I was slurring my words at the office long before I left for the 2:00 p.m. infusion.

Two sweet nurses, Melanie and Katrina hooked me up for the chemo and then kindly sat with me until the infusion was finished. "I knew you'd be all right," one of them said, disconnecting the I.V. just as Carla came by to see how things had gone.

"Nothing to report," I updated her. In fact, the Valium reaction was the only slightly unusual aspect of the whole shebang.

At home Dave and I ate dinner, watched a video, and went to bed. All routine follow-up to my Friday treatment. I didn't sense any nausea, but I didn't want to push it, either, so I opted to hold off on my bath until the next morning. I guess it was just the sensation of the chemo in my body that made me a bit cautious.

I woke up at 2:00 a.m. and took a preemptive Zofran—to "stay ahead of it" I reasoned. Later on I took a second one. Fine. No problems so far. When Dave came in to wake me and said that it was 10:30 I could hardly believe my ears. I felt okay and figured I could handle some breakfast. Toast, a banana, some orange juice.

It went down fine. And in less than an hour it came back up—hard! I ran to the bathroom when the impulse to vomit hit me. Dave followed and wrapped his arms around me for support as I let it go. The puking kept up all day long, starting the whole big negative spiral. What a letdown! Just after my bland breakfast, I had treated myself to the delightful thought that maybe this time I'd done it—that I'd get by without any of this junk.

The nausea and vomiting continued and caused me to slip quickly into a state of dehydration and weakness. Recognizing the familiar danger signs, Dave whisked me to the hospital for treatment, where I spent the rest of the weekend. The episode was a real blow to my health and my cancer-fighting ego!

A week after my discharge from the hospital I had a tap—the kind that draws fluid from around the lungs to ease the build-up of pressure. As always, at first I rejected any notion of further intrusion into this scar-covered body, but then gave in to the medical facts of life that stared me in the eyes, particularly the one that kept me from drawing a full breath.

During the tap procedure Dave and Carla looked on and we all talked. At one point they mentioned to the doctor that I am, indeed, Miss Ovarian Cancer, though unofficial and uncrowned. We began to laugh. I was quickly and sternly told that I'd need to be perfectly still or risk puncturing my right lung with the needle that was slowly withdrawing the menacing fluid. I could hear Dave and Carla commenting on how fast the yellow-colored fluid was draining into its container behind me.

While I got some relief from the fluid tap, the doctor was only able to drain part of the fluid because I started coughing—a natural consequence of the procedure. As fluid drains away and provides more room for the lung, it tries to inflate, attempting to expand to its normal size. This expansion creates a tickling sensation and then a coughing reflex. I tried to stifle them, but couldn't, so the thoracic surgeon had to stop the procedure or risk damaging my lung with the needle.

I asked to see the stuff that had been interfering with my breathing. I was amazed at the volume! It was about 450 cc's, enough to fill a sixteen ounce soda bottle! Next I had an "expiratory X-ray"—a picture of the lungs after I've just exhaled a deep breath.

"There's still some fluid there," said the surgeon, "But overall, your lungs look okay." And with that, Dave went after the car and Carla wheeled me out to the sidewalk where I breathed in the warm air of a Friday afternoon.

I was encouraged with the outcome of the day and returned home to spend the weekend with my husband, our dog, my comfortable bed and the good old yellow food menu, crossing my fingers and praying that I'd weather this unexpected summer storm.

This Too, Shall Pass

My recent extended bout of chemo complications and general malaise brought about my longest absence from work since the days of heavy-duty vertigo. I could do nothing. People stayed with me for the first week to cook and help get my meals. Carla and a friend from work even took a day off to help me out.

Eventually I got strong enough to fix my own meals, or Dave prepared them and came home at noon to heat them up. During that down period someone always came to pick me up for my lab tests at the hospital, and any other appointments I needed to keep.

On Monday, July 9th, I returned to work for the first time since early June when the bad chemo knocked me on my butt. I was determined to make it through that first week back on the job. People suggested I work a half-week, take it easy, and make a gradual move back to the office. Instead I followed my own rules.

Monday went okay. On Tuesday morning I went in to work early, at about seven. Somewhere around noon I started developing some pain in my abdomen. As the afternoon went on it got worse and worse. I was meeting with my boss and I didn't want to leave before we finished, around 5:30.

When I got home I was nearly in tears because the pain had gotten so much worse. Dave pulled into the garage just before me, so I asked him to grab my purse off the front seat.

"I can't lift it for some reason," I said.

"What's wrong?" he wanted to know.

"I'm not sure, but something's definitely wrong." I went straight upstairs to the bedroom, took off my work clothes and lay on my stomach thinking about what could be causing this pain. It hurt so much and seemed to be getting worse. The pain quickly became excruciating. I broke out in a cold sweat, followed by a chill at around 8:00 p.m. Then I started throwing up, even though I was not nauseated. I knew it was the terrible pain that was causing me to vomit.

Around midnight it started to ease. Dave gave me one of his stern, "You're not going in to work!" warnings. But I was so determined to make it through the week that I drove myself there and "walked" in, albeit humped over. A friend asked me what was wrong and all I could say was, "I'm not sure, but this is the most horrible pain I've ever had." It still hurt—to the point that I couldn't even put my fingers on my stomach without causing more discomfort. At some point I realized I'd forgotten to go to the hospital that day to have my regular blood labs drawn for chemo. A friend from work volunteered to drive me there, but by the time we arrived I could barely walk in the door and up to the lab. When we returned to the office, the pain started letting up. I stayed seated at my desk until it was time to leave work.

At home I picked up a Federal Express package waiting on the front porch steps. I noticed with interest that the return address was the Salt Lake City Olympic Committee. My mind raced, what in the world could this be? I unzipped the package and read the words, "Congratulations! You've been selected to carry the Olympic torch." I was thrilled! "I get to carry an OLYMPIC TORCH!" I proclaimed to no one but Winston and me.

Julie Lattanzi, a friend at work, had told me two weeks earlier that she'd sent a nomination to the committee, explaining why I had become her inspiration, but I really hadn't given the nomination any more serious thought until this moment.

In typical Nancy Lofstead fashion, the excitement turned to a brief wave of panic. What if I can't walk? After all, I'd been so sick I'd had to ride in a wheelchair at the last Relay for Life just weeks before. How can I carry a torch? Will I be strong enough? I was reading through the paperwork as more thoughts came to mind. I could wear my Miss Ovarian Cancer banner, wear my warm-up suit, hold *Nancy's Journey* in one hand and carry the torch in the other.

Then a few practical, more immediate concerns took over my concentration. I let Winston out, walked to the mailbox at the curb to see what other news might be awaiting me, and then went inside to use the bathroom. When I finished and stood up I noticed blood in the toilet. I stared at it for a moment or two, thinking out loud, "Hmmm, that's not good. I'll have to call the doctor."

It was almost 5:00 so she'd already left for the day. I told my story to a nurse practitioner instead. Without hesitation she said, "And I suppose you've been at work today?"

"Yes, I've been at work," I admitted.

She said I should go to the hospital because a kidney stone was likely. Dave was in Pittsburgh that day on business, so I couldn't call him to accompany me. I didn't want to scare Dad. Linda next door was not home, nor was my sister-in-law, Becky. Out of habit, I picked up the phone and called Carla.

"Carla, I'm passing blood in my urine and the doctor's office has told me to go to the E.R."

Predictably, she said, "I'm on my way."

I figured I'd better call Dad at that point and let him know what was up, because if he phoned and got no answer he'd be worried that something had happened during my first week back in the office.

When I told Dad that Carla was picking me up, he sounded surprised. "Isn't today the day she's leaving for her vacation in Ohio?"

I kicked myself for forgetting this important detail and wished I hadn't bothered her, throwing off her family travel plans. She ended up sitting in the emergency room with me from 5:00 till 9:00. The doctor ordered my blood chemistry, along with a urinalysis, which showed there was still plenty of blood present.

I'd reached Dave on his cell phone and began to tell him what had happened, in a good-news, bad-news jingle. The good news is I'm going to be an Olympic torchbearer! And the bad news? Can you meet me at the hospital?"

He came directly to the hospital. "Are you guys hungry?" he asked us, almost as soon as he arrived.

"I'm starving," I said. He drove to a nearby restaurant and got us some sandwiches. We ate. We waited. There had been so many slightly similar scenarios in the past, it was hard to tell what the verdict might be this time. At close to 9:00 we were told I probably had a bacterial infection in my urinary tract. This is one serious U.T.I. I thought to myself!

Okay, I can deal with a U.T.I. I started taking the Cipro antibiotic the E.R. doctor had prescribed for me. Still, I was bothered by the question, "How could a U.T.I. have caused all that pain?"

I got up the next morning and went to work. Shortly after I got situated at my desk, I started running to the bathroom with diarrhea. I phoned my primary care doctor who was aware that I'd called in the night before.

"Apparently I can't tolerate the Cipro," I told her.

"Just a minute, I'm going to go check the results of your urine culture." The doctor informed me the lab culture did not indicate a U.T.I. She said, "You can quit the antibiotic. It's probably not a tract infection that's making you sick. I think it was a kidney stone—and you passed it before the bleeding started. Get an I.V.P. at the hospital on Saturday."

The I.V.P. (intravenous pyelogram) is a test that involves being injected with a dye to let doctors observe the flow from the kidneys down through the urinary tract, monitoring for any abnormalities. I followed her instructions and had the I.V.P. performed that weekend. Everything came back clean, no stones were found, but it took several days for my intestines to recover from the Cipro.

By Monday my tummy was no longer tender. That next week back at work went better, and the following was better still. I wasn't going to give in. I'd been determined to survive that first week and set the tone for my re-entry. It gave me a real sense of accomplishment to be there those first five days in a row. Kidney stone? No big deal. I have cancer. I just wanted to get back to the clinic and do my job. Kidney stones are normal, run-of-the-mill things, the kind of problem that happens to other people. Kidney stones are not on my list of reasons to miss work. Cancer is, but not kidney stones, oh, and maybe hives, if they're bad enough!

It's Allllllways Something!

In the course of being off work during this last bout, my doctor suggested I try to reintroduce the enzyme I'd been using to help me with my chronic diarrhea problem. It's supposed to make up for my poor, worn-out liver's inability to produce the enzyme for me naturally and help my system absorb nutrients and fat. I started out taking the enzyme in three separate doses on the first day. And in no time—whammo!—I'd broken out in hives! One ear turned blood red and there were bright splotches all over my neck. I pulled up my nightgown the next morning to find the rash all over my chest.

My doctor's advice? "Take some Benadryl. If you're not clear by morning, come in."

I downed the Benadryl. It made me so drowsy I almost fell asleep in my plate at dinner that evening. The hives were worse the next day. I've often relied on Dad and on Linda next door for getting me to the hospital to have my labs drawn and this freaky episode was no exception. Linda drove me to the doctor's office, telling me along the route to sit on my hands and please try not to scratch. I couldn't wait for whatever relief was available to me.

It took a strong anti-histamine to counteract the unusual allergic response to the enzyme, which means I had to wait a bit before I attempted to start the enzyme regimen again. My primary care doctor had hoped I could get back on track with the enzyme supplement and start weaning myself off the tincture of opium I've taken for the chronic diarrhea for almost a year now. It seems with the kidney stone, and then the hives, that I simply can't get back on a regular schedule—can't even get to the starting line to take off in the race!

Never mind kidney stones and hives. At this point, just putting on a few pounds would make me feel like a success story. Weight loss has been a serious problem for me, beginning with a gradual decrease that's held on since late last fall. I normally weigh around 125 to 128 pounds. My oncologist has said I shouldn't go below 115 (I'm a whopping 111 and holding, but just barely—down two pounds from last month). At one point he wanted me to start on a nutritional food supplement that's administered through an I.V. in my port. The thought of it is repulsive to me and I quickly let him know I wouldn't be agreeing to that alternative any time soon.

Besides, I eat three meals a day plus a snack. I just don't feel I truly have the capacity for a lot of food, at least not consumed all at once. I feel full *while* I'm eating. It's probably because there are tumors pressing on my stomach. Because I can't eat three huge meals a day, I try to eat small quantities at a time and then follow up with a bit more food about an hour after my meal. There's even my daily ice cream protocol. I eat a Dairy Queen Dilly Bar nearly every night, the kind our local D.Q. makes according to my special order to try and help me fatten up—chocolate ice cream *and* chocolate shell! I like the D.Q. Blizzards as well, but because they're so rich, I have to be concerned about diarrhea.

Everyone's got an opinion on the weight matter. They're always saying, "Eat this. Eat that." The dietician on our staff has been very helpful to me. She's given me some good tips about drinking fruit juices, snacking, and so on. I continue to take the tincture of opium I've been relying on since last fall. It helps me manage the chronic diarrhea I've had for the past few years now. It even lets me eat a wider range of foods when I'm feeling good— my beloved chocolate, for instance.

With all of this, I still can't gain any weight. It's so difficult and frustrating. I think it's probably just as bad to be thin and trying unsuccessfully to gain weight as to be heavy and not able to lose. I'm really struggling to get my weight back, but for now I have to be content with maintaining what I've got and gaining minute amounts at infrequent intervals. If I'm lucky, maybe I can add a few pounds before our upcoming Sisters' Weekend, or at the very latest, by the time I appear "in" the 2002 Winter Olympics!

I'm so excited. That is one BIG CARROT dangling out there! And I can't even talk out loud about it! Because the Olympic folks haven't yet released the news of the torchbearer selections to the media, I'm not allowed to tell anyone other than immediate family members. At the same time, I'm really hoping to get pumped up. We torchbearers can't be showing up with little chicken legs and risk embarrassing the entire country on ESPN. I also want to bulk up my arms so I can hold that torch just as high as any of the other participants.

With these very objectives in mind, I *did* break down and tell my boss John about the Olympic deal because I had to start preparing. He put some of the Clinic's athletic trainers and physical therapists in charge of my strength and conditioning program. Believe me, with my body, which must seem a bit like the MIR Space Station with its multiple scars and patches, they've got a challenge ahead of them. The gang suspects I have some ulterior motives in my new fitness quest, they just don't know yet what those motives are!

I'll be part of the relay that wraps through West Virginia and Pennsylvania. Three weeks before the December event I'm supposed to get a letter telling exactly when and where I'll be carrying the torch. I do know it will be on either a Wednesday or Thursday, so I'll probably have to sneak out of work.

I've already filled out all the necessary Olympic forms. I had to choose how I would complete my two-tenths of a mile segment: walker, wheelchair, walk, brisk walk, or run. I checked "walk." There weren't any "other" categories for roller blades or bikes. I should probably attempt a couple laps around Mountaineer Field to get my gears in motion.

They'll also be sending me the outfit I'm supposed to wear: 1) an official Olympic long-sleeved, crew-neck shirt; 2) a jogging suit; and 3) a fleece hat and gloves. They're leaving the choice of footwear up to me.

I have to try and stay focused on today just so I don't go crazy counting down the days until December. I feel like a little kid on Christmas Eve who won't be able to sleep if I really start thinking about the excitement ahead. Besides, managing my next round of chemo is akin to my own personal Olympics.

The Value of Work

I pride myself in the fact that, despite all the pitfalls of the last dozen years, my overall work attendance has not been too shabby. I doubt that anyone would have been able to distinguish my record of total sick days from the average Joe's, at least until now.

This last struggle kept me off work for five weeks—the longest chunk of time I've missed since the vertigo problem leveled me back in '97. In each of these five weeks, there didn't seem to be even one day when I thought I could make it in to the office. Physically, I could barely get up and go. I began to entertain the question, "Why go back?" In a call to my Baltimore oncologist's office I mentioned my deep frustration to my old pal Barb, who still works as a secretary there.

She knows me fairly well after all these years and had been worried about me during the recent long period of illness, but she wanted nothing to do with the notion I might not make it back to work. Barb said she was afraid for me, "If we take your job away you'll lose your focus."

I argued with her. "So you expect me to keep working?"

"Nancy," she said, "We see 120 cancer patients in this clinic and not one of them works! You're not like them. *You're* not the normal cancer patient." She thought maybe I was finally reaching the point the other patients had already gotten to—feeling unable to maintain a career or employment—many of them were probably on total disability status.

I was getting more defensive as the conversation continued, "Yeah? Well maybe *they're* not normal. Maybe *I'm* the only normal one in the bunch! Maybe I've started to lose ground in this thing. Maybe it's time for me to hang it up, just quit work and stay at home."

I began to cry and I sensed she was getting emotional too. We ended the phone call on a sad note. After a couple days had passed and I felt more in control, I phoned her back to apologize and talk some more.

"Are you doing better today?" Barb asked.

I can be honest with her. We've known each other for so long and she's seen me go through a lot over time. "Yup. I'm okay," I answered, feeling a bit more collected.

I'd been thinking it over. Barb was right about one thing. Without my job to lend some structure to each week, I *had* begun to lose my focus. It's normal to work, as far as Nancy's Rules go. Dragging my butt in there at times when I didn't feel well was the right step for me. Not that I'm tough, it's more because work is my link to survival. It lets me focus on a professional agenda rather than on a cancer agenda. Maybe it wouldn't benefit others, but it does help me. It's important. Besides, my emotional health gets a boost when I have more interaction.

For me, the workplace is a family setting. With my office family I've always felt as though I had this circle around me so that if I faltered or started to lean, someone would catch me or help brace me up. And it's true. Someone *is* always there. Someone always catches me. They're my support team.

I feel so fortunate compared to many of the cancer patients I meet. A lot of them don't have the support network that family, church, and good co-workers can provide. When that's the case, cancer patients typically withdraw. I don't plan to behave in a typical way.

I want to associate with positive people—it's part of fighting the battle. You can't hold an illness at bay, and you certainly can't conquer it, if you're carrying a bunch of negativity around, blaming someone or something for your unhappiness. I'm determined to expend my limited energy in a positive direction. The blessing of a great support group at work helps me do just that.

I used this positive energy rationale when I went back on the 5 FU after my run-in with the Carboplatin and when I began feeling better physically. I thought, by golly, *this* buckaroo is FINALLY recovering from the aftermath. I knew my mind and body needed to "get back in the saddle" and resume my office routine. There was no pressure from anyone at the clinic to return, but the mental focus a schedule can offer was just what I needed.

The Here and Now

Once again I find myself waiting impatiently for a perfect chemo. One that won't make me so sick. One that will squelch the hungry trouble brewing in me. My side is protruding from a tumor that's demanding its elbowroom in my ribcage. South of that, crowding outward from the cradle of my pelvis, is a lump that looks like a couple marbles I might have swallowed as a kid. And there are more. It's clear my body has become a harbor for the "Big C's" enemy fleet. I try not to dwell on the persistent question my conscience has begun to ask, "Will I know when I've simply had enough?"

It is summer once again in Morgantown. The trees in our back yard have formed a thick, shady curtain between our place and the lower hillside. The potted plants on our deck are green and lush, thriving in the sultry air. Ignoring the season, my Christmas cactus just surprised me and sprouted a darling little blossom. And the other day a butterfly I'd never met landed on the porch for a breather. She was a beautiful weave of silver and gold and as big as a slice of warm toast.

The streets have been swept free of the excess traffic the university calendar draws. The downtown sidewalks breathe a bit more easily minus a few thousand pedestrians schlepping backpacks from coffee shop to class.

The August weather hugs the hillsides on its way to the river, shrouding them in a hazy, visible warmth. Stand on any street corner and you're bound to hear what we've all known since the day summer was created, "It's not the heat. It's the humidity. That's what gets ya!" If only it were that simple.

⚭

The journey continues.